OVERVIEW MAP KEY

:: OTHER TITLES IN THIS SERIES

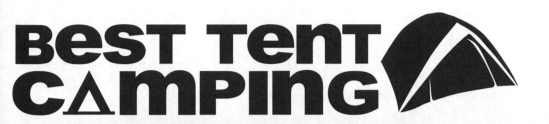

BEST TENT CAMPING

WEST VIRGINIA

YOUR CAR-CAMPING GUIDE TO SCENIC BEAUTY, THE SOUNDS OF NATURE, AND AN ESCAPE FROM CIVILIZATION

3rd Edition

JOHNNY MOLLOY

MENASHA RIDGE PRESS
Your Guide to the Outdoors Since 1982

:: *This book is for my longtime West Virginia friend, Steve Grayson.*

Best Tent Camping: West Virginia, 3rd Edition

Copyright © 2014 by Johnny Molloy
All rights reserved
Printed in the United States of America
Published by Menasha Ridge Press
Distributed by Publishers Group West
Third edition, first printing

Library of Congress Cataloging-in-Publication Data
Molloy, Johnny, 1961-
  Best tent camping : West Virginia : your car camping guide to scenic beauty, the sounds
of nature, and an escape from civilization / Johnny Molly. -- Third edition.
     pages cm. -- (Best tent camping)
  Distributed by the Publishers' Group West.
  ISBN 978-0-89732-495-3 (paperback) -- ISBN 0-89732-495-1 (paperback) --
ISBN 978-0-89732-497-7 (eBook)
  1. Camping--West Virginia--Guidebooks. 2. Camp sites, facilities, etc.--West Virginia
--Directories. 3. West Virginia--Guidebooks. I. Title.
  GV191.42.W4M64 2014
  796.5409754--dc23
                              2014013211

Cover design by Scott McGrew
Cover photo by Joseph Sohm
Text design by Annie Long
Cartography by Steve Jones and Johnny Molloy
Indexing by Rich Carlson

Menasha Ridge Press
An imprint of Keen Communications, LLC
P.O. Box 43673
Birmingham, Alabama 35243
menasharidge.com

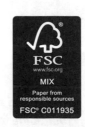

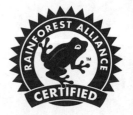

FSC
www.fsc.org
MIX
Paper from
responsible sources
FSC® C011935

CONTENTS

● ● ● ● ● ● ● ● ● ● ● ● ● ● ● ● ● ● ● ●

:: ALLEGHENY HIGHLANDS 9

:: EASTERN PANHANDLE 58

BEST CAMPGROUNDS

● ●

ACKNOWLEDGMENTS

● ●

I would like to thank the following people for helping me in the research and writing of this book: Keri Anne Molloy, Robert and Bonnie Gross, Roxanna Carr, Roy Reynolds, Jat Hedrick, Anna Galenza at Bulltown, Karen Stokes, Cindy Thomas, Mike Foster, and Cindy Blair. Thanks to Frank Sellars for his information on the New River, and to Stephanie Bailey and Barbara Breshock for getting questioned during their lunch. Thanks to John Markwell at the Gendarme in Seneca Rocks for his advice about the area. Thanks to Dale A. Porter for his books and information. Thanks to Keith Stinnett, Deal Holcomb, Cisco Meyer, Nelle Molloy, Steele Molloy, and Pat Molloy.

Thanks to Kelty for providing me with excellent tents, backpacks, sleeping bags, and outerwear.

The biggest thanks of all goes to the people of West Virginia, who love their mountain lands.

PREFACE

● ●

Welcome to the third edition of *Best Tent Camping West Virginia*. Part of the fun of updating this book is the excuse it gives me to go tent camping in the Mountain State yet again. With a Jeep, a laptop computer, and an open mind, I set forth into the hills of West Virginia. The first trip started in the spring. In southwest West Virginia, historic coal country, I came upon my first surprise, Panther Wildlife Management Area. The place was covered in wildflowers! It started raining the next morning. Such are times that a tent camper has to face. Next I headed up the Ohio River Valley. Amid the development along the waterway, I found other gems, such as Tomlinson Run, where the trees of the hilltop campground hadn't begun to leaf out and where I spent a cold night as the sole occupant of the campground.

More trips extended into the summer. As the weather warmed in the "lowlands" around me, the Alleghenies and lake areas became the places to go. The weather was great and the scenery even better. Getaways like Bulltown, an Army Corps of Engineers preserve, offered a watery place to cool off, as well as glimpses into the vast human history of the Mountain State. Other times I headed high into the Monongahela National Forest, to places like Bear Heaven, where on July evenings I donned a jacket and scooted a little closer to the campfire.

The more campgrounds I visited, the more I appreciated the people who operated these preserves. They were hardworking, enthusiastic patrons of their lands. Sometimes a great park staff was saddled with a mediocre campground, and it was disappointing not to be able to include them.

The days began to shorten—fall was on its way. There were still more campgrounds to inspect, and I headed down to the New River area. I had rafted that river, as well as the Gauley, in previous years and knew how scenic these gorges were. I enjoyed Glade Creek, part of the New River National Recreation Area, so much I went back for a second visit under the guise of "making sure" it should be in the book.

And with the joy of completing a book and the sadness of an adventure ended, I finished my research. But, not surprisingly, within a month of turning in the original manuscript, I returned with a friend to the Dolly Sods for a backpacking trip and to the upper New River for a canoe trip. And so I have returned to the Mountain State for years since the first edition and second edition, going on adventures, staying in the campgrounds again, and writing about them. May you have many return adventures of your own.

INTRODUCTION

● ●

How to Use This Guidebook

The publishers of Menasha Ridge Press welcome you to *Best Tent Camping West Virginia*. Whether you're new to this activity or you've been sleeping in your portable outdoor shelter over decades of outdoor adventures, please review the following information. It explains how we have worked with the author to organize this book and how you can make the best use of it.

Some passages in this introduction are applicable to all of the books in the Best Tent Camping guidebook series. Where this isn't the case, such as in the descriptions of weather, wildlife, and plants, the author has provided information specific to your area.

:: THE RATINGS & RATING CATEGORIES

Included in this book is a rating system for West Virginia's 50 best tent campgrounds. Certain campground attributes—beauty, privacy, spaciousness, quiet, security, and cleanliness—are ranked using a star system. Five stars are ideal; one is acceptable. This system will help you find the campground that has the attributes you desire. Below and following, we describe the criteria for each of the attributes in our five-star rating system:

★ ★ ★ ★ ★   The site is **ideal** in that category.

★ ★ ★ ★   The site is **exemplary** in that category.

★ ★ ★   The site is **very good** in that category.

★ ★   The site is **above average** in that category.

★   The site is **acceptable** in that category.

Beauty

In the best campgrounds, the fluid shapes and elements of nature—flora, water, land, and sky—have melded to create locales that seem to have been made for tent camping. The best sites are so attractive you may be tempted not to leave your outdoor home. A little site work is all right to make the scenic area camper-friendly, but too many reminders of civilization eliminated many a campground from inclusion in this book.

Privacy

A little understory goes a long way in making you feel comfortable once you've picked your site for the night. There is a trend to plant natural borders between campsites if the borders don't exist already. With some trees or brush to define the sites, everyone has personal space. Then you can go about the pleasures of tent camping without keeping up with the Joneses at the site next door—or them with you.

Spaciousness

This attribute can be very important, depending on how much of a gearhead you are and the size of your group. Campers with family-style tents need to have a large, flat spot on which to pitch their tent and still be able to get to the ice chest to prepare food, while not getting burned near the fire ring. Gearheads need adequate space to show off all their stuff to neighbors strolling by. I just want enough room to keep my bedroom, den, and kitchen separate.

Quiet

The music of the mountains—the singing birds, rushing streams, windblown meadows and trees—includes the kinds of noises tent campers associate with being in West Virginia. In concert, they camouflage the sounds you don't want to hear—autos coming and going, loud neighbors, and so on.

Security

Campground security is relative. A remote campground is usually safe, but don't tempt potential thieves by leaving your valuables out for all to see. Use common sense, and go with your instinct. Campground hosts are wonderful to have around, and state parks with locked gates are ideal for security. Get to know your neighbors, and develop a buddy system to watch each other's belongings when possible.

Cleanliness

I'm a stickler for this one. Nothing sabotages a scenic campground like trash. Most of the campgrounds in this guidebook are clean. More rustic campgrounds—my favorites—usually receive less maintenance. Busy weekends and holidays will show their effects; however, don't let a little litter spoil your good time. Help clean up, and think of it as doing your part for West Virginia's natural environment.

:: THE CAMPGROUND PROFILE

Each profile contains a concise but informative narrative of the campground and individual sites. Not only is the property described, but readers can also get a general idea of the recreational opportunities available—what's in the area and perhaps suggestions for touristy activities. This descriptive text is enhanced with three helpful sidebars: Ratings, Key Information, and Getting There (accurate driving directions that lead you to the campground from the nearest major roadway, along with GPS coordinates).

:: THE OVERVIEW MAP, MAP KEY, AND LEGEND

Use the overview map on the inside front cover to assess the exact location of each campground. The campground's number appears not only on the overview map but also on the map key facing the overview map, in the table of contents, and on the profile's first page. This book is organized by region, as indicated in the table of contents.

A map legend that details the symbols found on the campground-layout maps appears on the inside back cover.

:: CAMPGROUND-LAYOUT MAPS

Each profile includes a detailed map of campground sites, internal roads, facilities, and other key items.

:: GPS CAMPGROUND-ENTRANCE COORDINATES

Readers can easily access all campgrounds in this book by using the directions given and the overview map, which shows at least one major road leading into the area. But for those who enjoy using GPS technology to navigate, the book includes coordinates for each campground's entrance in latitude and longitude, expressed in degrees and decimal minutes. To convert GPS coordinates from degrees, minutes, and seconds to the above degrees–decimal minutes format, the seconds are divided by 60. For more on GPS technology, visit **usgs.gov.**

A note of caution: Actual GPS devices will easily guide you to any of these campgrounds, but users of smartphone mapping apps will find that cell phone service is often unavailable in the hills and hollows where many of these hideaways are located.

About This Book

West Virginia is an unusual state. Born of the Civil War, culled from the Old Dominion, it has been called the northernmost Southern state, or the southernmost Northern state. Its nickname is the Mountain State, and mountainous it is. It has been said that if the ridges and peaks of West Virginia were flattened out, it would be the size of Texas. With straight roads and flat lands few and far between, it has the highest average elevation of any state east of the Mississippi River.

I call it the most untapped natural resource in the East. In fact, the entire state of West Virginia deserves to be a National Park. It is that beautiful. Nevertheless, progress and people came (not always a bad thing) and settled what was then Old Virginia, building lives and communities in hollows along the streams and rivers. West Virginia became a state, and special places began to be set aside for nature to dominate.

Today, tent campers can enjoy these parcels, pieces of each distinct region of West Virginia. In Feudin' Country, named after the infamous Hatfield–McCoy quarrels of yesteryear, you can explore the hilliest terrain of the Mountain State, or any other state, for that matter. The Ohio River Valley is the land of frontiersmen and American Indians, where history played out as the human tide swept westward. The New River Valley is home to one of the continent's oldest rivers, which has cut a scenic swath through the ridges of coal country. The Heart of West Virginia is a region of lakes, where numerous reservoirs offer water recreation. The Allegheny Highlands have the highest elevations and most diverse forests, crowned with dark stands of red spruce. The Eastern Panhandle has the drier pine/oak/hickory highlands interspersed with rock outcrops, offering scenic views of valleys below.

All this spells paradise for the tent camper. No matter where you go, the scenery will never fail to please. Before embarking on a trip, take time to prepare. Many of the best tent campgrounds are a fair distance from the civilized world, and you want to enjoy yourself rather than make supply or gear runs. Call ahead and ask for a park map, brochure, or other information to help you plan your trip. Visit the campground's or park's website. Make reservations wherever possible, especially at popular state parks. Do research. Ask questions. The more you ask, the fewer surprises you'll find. There are other times, however, when you'll just want to grab your gear and this book, hop in the car, and wing it.

If traveling to the Monongahela National Forest, call ahead and order a forest map, or purchase one online through their website. The phone number is 304-636-1800. Not only will a map make it that much easier to reach your destination, but nearby hikes, scenic drives, waterfalls, and landmarks will also be easier to find. There are forest visitor centers in addition to ranger stations. Call or visit, and ask questions. When ordering a map, ask for any additional literature about the area in which you are interested.

In writing this book, I had the pleasure of meeting many friendly, helpful people: local residents proud of their West Virginia mountains, along with state park and national forest employees who endured my endless questions. Even better were my fellow tent campers, who were eager to share their knowledge about their favorite spots. They already know what a lovely place West Virginia is. As the splendor of the Mountain State becomes more recognized, these lands become that much more precious. Enjoy them, protect them, and use them wisely.

:: WEATHER

West Virginia offers four distinct seasons, although Mother Nature sometimes gets them confused. In short, year-round camping is a real possibility, but extreme winter weather will be more likely and severe the higher you go in elevation. Summer is often hot and humid, but the rivers, swimming holes, and lakes at most campgrounds keep campers comfortable in even the worst heat wave. Spring and fall are ideal times to be outdoors in West Virginia. In spring, wildflowers are everywhere, dogwood and redwood blooms brighten the forest, and spring peepers serenade you from the lakes and streams near camp. Fall in the mountains is nearly everyone's favorite camping season. Cold frosty mornings chip away at the lassitude left from summer's heat. In fall's crisp air, you begin breathing easily and deeply for the first time in months, and your body wakes up ready to hit the trails. Hues of orange, red, yellow, and caramel decorate the forest as the trees prepare to shed their summer foliage. Additional benefits of autumn camping are the absence of humidity, heat, bugs, and crowds; the streams are shallow and easier to cross; and the bare trees open up scenic views obscured by lush foliage during the warmer months.

:: FIRST-AID KIT

A useful first-aid kit may contain more items than you might think necessary. These are just the basics. Prepackaged kits in waterproof bags (Atwater Carey and Adventure Medical make them) are available. As a preventive measure, take along sunscreen and insect repellent. Even though quite a few items are listed here, they pack down into a small space:

- Ace bandages or Spenco joint wraps
- Adhesive bandages, such as Band-Aids
- Antibiotic ointment (Neosporin or the generic equivalent)
- Antiseptic or disinfectant, such as Betadine or hydrogen peroxide
- Aspirin, acetaminophen, or ibuprofen
- Benadryl or the generic equivalent, diphenhydramine (in case of allergic reactions)
- Butterfly-closure bandages
- Comb and tweezers (for removing ticks from your skin)
- Epinephrine in a prefilled syringe (for severe allergic reactions to such things as bee stings)
- Gauze (one roll and six 4-by-4-inch compress pads
- LED flashlight or headlamp
- Matches or lighter
- Moist towlettes
- Moleskin/Spenco 2nd Skin
- Pocketknife or multipurpose tool
- Waterproof first-aid tape
- Whistle (it's more effective in signaling rescuers than your voice)

:: ANIMAL AND PLANT HAZARDS

Bears

Ursus Americanus, the American Black Bear, was reintroduced into Arkansas around 1960. They are not uncommon in West Virginia's mountains. Normal precautions for keeping nuisance animals, such as raccoons and opossums, out of your food supply are usually all that's necessary when camping. Check campground bulletin boards when you pull into camp—there will be a notice posted if recent bear activity has occurred in the camp or its surrounding area, along with additional precautions you should take. In areas with high bear activity, be sure to use specially designed food containers. Never keep food in your tent.

Poison Ivy

This little three-leaf villain is common throughout West Virginia. Watch for its three-leaf configuration, both in ground cover and vines on trees near your campsite. Within 14 hours of exposure, you'll have blisters and a terrible itch in the affected area. Wash and dry the area thoroughly with alcohol, soap, and cold water as soon as possible after exposure. Wearing long pants and sleeves will help protect you, but be careful—touching your clothing or even pets or camping gear that have contacted poison ivy may spread the plant's rash-producing oil onto your skin. If you're sensitive to the ivy's effects, bring along one of the various over-the-counter products that alleviate poison ivy's irritating symptoms.

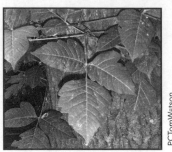

Snakes

Venomous snakes aren't a huge problem in West Virginia, but they're out there. Copperheads are the most common. Timber rattlesnakes are occasionally sighted in the mountains. You may spot snakes in streams, lakes, and even in pools along trails in the campgrounds. Unless they're torpid from cold weather, snakes will see you or sense your footfalls before you reach them and most likely move away.

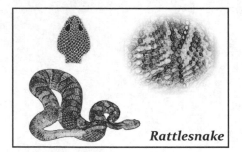

Rattlesnake

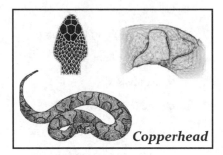

Copperhead

Ticks

Ticks are ubiquitous throughout West Virginia, especially in warmer months. You can contract Lyme disease and Rocky Mountain spotted fever from these annoying little critters, but it rarely happens, especially if you're vigilant and remove them soon after they find you. Wearing light-colored clothing makes them easier to spot, and an insect repellent with DEET helps keep them away. Ticks prefer places where they're held tightly against your skin, such as elastic on socks and underwear, your underarms, waistband, and back of the knee. Tweezers are ideal for removing a tick that has already attached—just grab it as close to the skin surface as possible and firmly pull it loose without crushing it. Expect a bit of redness and itching for a few days around the bite site.

:: CAMPING ETIQUETTE

Here are a few tips on how to create good vibes with fellow campers and wildlife you encounter.

- Make sure that you check in, pay your fee, and mark your site as directed. Don't make the mistake of grabbing a seemingly empty site that looks more appealing than your site. It could be reserved. If you're unhappy with the site you've selected, check with the campground host for other options.

- Be sensitive to the ground beneath you. Place all garbage in designated receptacles or pack it out if none is available. No one likes to see the trash that someone else has left behind.

- It's common for animals to wander through campsites, where they may be accustomed to the presence of humans (and our food). An unannounced approach, a sudden movement, or a loud noise startles most animals. A surprised animal can be dangerous to you, to others, and to themselves. Give them plenty of space.

- Plan ahead. Know your equipment, your ability, and the area where you are camping—and prepare accordingly. Be self-sufficient at all times; carry necessary supplies for changes in weather or other conditions. A well-executed trip is a satisfaction to you and to others.

- Be courteous to other campers, hikers, bikers, and anyone else you encounter.

- Strictly follow the campground's rules regarding the building of fires. Never burn trash. Trash smoke smells horrible, and trash debris in a fire pit or grill is unsightly.

- Everyone likes a fire, but bringing your own firewood from home is now frowned upon by most campground operators. Bringing in wood from out of the area could introduce pests that are harmful to the forest. Use deadfall found near your campsite or purchase wood at the camp store.

:: HAPPY CAMPING

There is nothing worse than a bad camping trip, especially because it is so easy to have a great time. To assist with making your outing a happy one, here are some pointers:

- Reserve your site in advance, especially if it's a weekend or a holiday, or if the campground is wildly popular. Many prime campgrounds require at least a six-month lead time on reservations. Check before you go.

- Pick your camping buddies wisely. A family trip is pretty straightforward, but you may want to reconsider including grumpy Uncle Fred, who doesn't like bugs, sunshine, or marshmallows. After you know who's going, make sure that everyone is on the same page regarding expectations of difficulty (amenities or the lack thereof, physical exertion, and so on), sleeping arrangements, and food requirements.

- Don't duplicate equipment, such as cooking pots and lanterns, among campers in your party. Carry what you need to have a good time, but don't turn the trip into a cross-country moving experience.

■ Dress for the season. Educate yourself on the temperature highs and lows of the specific part of the state you plan to visit. It may be warm at night in the summer in your backyard, but up in the mountains it will be quite chilly.

■ Pitch your tent on a level surface, preferably one covered with leaves, pine straw, or grass. Use a tarp or specially designed footprint to thwart ground moisture and to protect the tent floor. Do a little site maintenance, such as picking up the small rocks and sticks that can damage your tent floor and make sleep uncomfortable. If you have a separate tent rain fly but don't think you'll need it, keep it rolled up at the base of the tent, in case it starts raining at midnight.

■ Consider taking a sleeping pad if the ground makes you uncomfortable. Choose a pad that is full-length and thicker than you think you might need. This will not only keep your hips from aching on hard ground, but it will also help keep you warm. A wide range of thin, light, or inflatable pads is available at camping stores today, and these are a much better choice than home air mattresses, which conduct heat away from the body and tend to deflate during the night.

■ If you are not hiking in to a primitive campsite, there is no real need to skimp on food due to weight. Plan tasty meals and bring everything you will need to prepare, cook, eat, and clean up.

■ If you tend to use the bathroom multiple times at night, you should plan ahead. Leaving a warm sleeping bag and stumbling around in the dark to find the restroom—whether it be a pit toilet, a fully plumbed comfort station, or just the woods—is not fun. Keep a flashlight and any other accoutrements you may need by the tent door and know exactly where to head in the dark.

■ Standing dead trees and storm-damaged living trees can pose a real hazard to tent campers. (Foresters call these widow-makers for obvious reasons.) These trees may have loose or broken limbs that could fall at any time. When choosing a campsite or even just a spot to rest during a hike, look up.

Allegheny Highlands

1

Bear Heaven

The 20,000-acre Otter Creek Wilderness is just minutes away from this small, secluded campground with a great view.

Bear Heaven lies on a spur ridge high on Shavers Mountain outside Elkins. It can be pretty cool on summer nights. I can only imagine how cold it is during the shoulder seasons. Most tent campers will head up this way during the warmer months to enjoy a small, quiet campground tucked away on the back side of the Otter Creek Wilderness.

The Otter Creek drainage forms the centerpiece of this preserved national forest land. Mountain ridges are the borders, where spruce stands and bogs hold strong. Lower in the wilderness are tangles of rhododendron over which grow Northern hardwood species, such as cherry and yellow birch. This area was once logged, and many trails follow old railroad grades. In other areas, apple trees mark homesites long since abandoned. On the edge of this wilderness, Bear Heaven campground awaits your arrival.

What does this mean for you? It means a great place to explore the heart of natural West Virginia, where the woods are king. After a day's hiking and sightseeing, you can return to your ridgetop camp and reflect on the day's sights. (One of those observations will be what a fitting campground this is to be adjacent to the Otter Creek Wilderness. Another might literally be a lookout—from atop the jumbled rock outcrop near the campground picnic area, where you can gaze south over a sea of wooded ridges.)

Leave the spur road off Stuart Memorial Drive and enter Bear Heaven Recreation Area. To your right is the picnic area and rock outcrop. This spur ridge is level by mountain standards and covered in a Northern hardwood forest dominated by beech and cherry trees. The canopy thickens in summer, with an understory of sugar maple and striped maple. After the leaves fall, you can better see the numerous gray boulders strewn about the campground like toy blocks tossed around a room.

Three sites occupy the main road. Log borders keep campers where they ought to be. The campsites are dispersed and large, even though this spur ridge is narrow. There are winter views into the woods below. Some less-than-level sites have tent pads.

Entering a five-campsite loop, sites 4 and 5, the two prettiest and most used, are integrated into the boulder-dominated landscape. Swing around the loop and pass the final few campsites. This small campground has only eight units, offering the good and bad of small campgrounds: intimate yet easily packed with campers. Bear Heaven fills during midsummer weekends

:: Ratings

BEAUTY: ★ ★ ★ ★ ★
PRIVACY: ★ ★ ★
SPACIOUSNESS: ★ ★ ★ ★
QUIET: ★ ★ ★ ★ ★
SECURITY: ★ ★ ★
CLEANLINESS: ★ ★ ★ ★

:: Key Information

ADDRESS: Bear Heaven, P.O. Box 368, Parsons, WV 26287

OPERATED BY: U.S. Forest Service

CONTACT: 304-478-3251, www.fs.usda.gov/mnf

OPEN: Late April–November

SITES: 8

SITE AMENITIES: Picnic table, fire grate, lantern post

ASSIGNMENT: First come, first served; no reservations

REGISTRATION: Self-registration on-site

FACILITIES: Vault toilets

PARKING: At campsites only

FEE: $5 per night

ELEVATION: 3,600 feet

RESTRICTIONS:
- **Pets:** On leash only
- **Fires:** In fire grates only
- **Alcohol:** At campsites only
- **Vehicles:** None
- **Other:** 14-day stay limit

and traditional summer holidays. Any other time, you should have no problem getting a campsite.

There are no trails leaving directly from the campground, other than the short walk to the rock outcrop by the picnic area, but there is a whole wilderness just to the north. Less than a mile away, on Forest Service Road 303, which you passed on the way in, lies the main trailhead for the southern side of the Otter Creek Wilderness. The area's 20,000 acres of rocky ridges and rhododendron-lined creeks, along with its wildlife, have thrived under wilderness protection since 1975.

Here, you can start the upper end of the Otter Creek Trail. This 11-mile footpath is the backbone of the trail system. Several loop hikes can be made using a combination of trails. One circuit starts north down the Otter Creek Trail and turns right on the Mylius Gap Trail. Climb up to Mylius Gap;

then turn right on the Shavers Mountain Trail and follow it for 4.3 miles to the Hedrick Camp Trail. Turn right here and you'll soon intersect the Otter Creek Trail for a 9.4-mile loop.

Or start at the top of Otter Creek Trail and walk 4.4 miles down to Pothole Falls, Otter Creek's tallest fall. Then return the way you came. To stay in the high country, start at Alpena Gap near US 33 and walk out along the Shavers Mountain Trail.

Even as remote as Bear Heaven seems, the fully equipped town of Elkins is just 10 miles away, in case you need supplies or any civilized trappings. Between Elkins and Bear Heaven is the Bowden Fish Hatchery. If you have never visited a hatchery, check it out. There are fish of all sizes swimming in the tanks. It may inspire you to take a rod down to Otter Creek and toss a line for the native brook trout lying secretively in the cool pools.

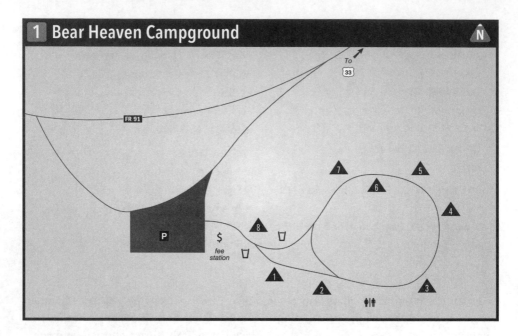

:: Getting There

From Elkins, drive east on US 33 for 11.5 miles to Stuart Memorial Drive (FR 91) at Alpena Gap on Shavers Mountain. Turn left on FR 91 and follow it 1.1 miles; then veer left, staying on FR 91. Continue on FR 91 for 1.5 miles to Bear Heaven Campground, which will be on your left.

GPS COORDINATES   N38° 55.841'   W79° 40.827'

2

Bishop Knob

Bishop Knob is a value for all tent campers.

Bishop **Knob** is an underutilized resource of the Monongahela National Forest. Other nearby campgrounds draw the crowds, leaving Bishop Knob to languish in obscurity. Don't pass this place by—and for eight bucks, what have you got to lose? Especially considering the assets of Bishop Knob and the other attractions that draw campers to the more popular campgrounds nearby.

So what's at Bishop Knob? Try a secluded and quiet ridgetop camping area with a few trails of its own and quick access to both the Williams and Cranberry Rivers. Plus, Bishop Knob rarely exceeds 50% capacity, which means you can nab a campsite already rife with natural privacy and make it even more private by having no one on either side of you. I stayed here on a Saturday in July with nary a soul within five campsites of me in any direction.

Situated in a dense hardwood forest of maple and oak, the 55 campsites are divided between two loops. Turn left into the first loop. The gravel road is wide, and the campsites are spread far apart. Thick undergrowth gives the level areas a greater sense of privacy, and mown edges along the

gravel road and campsites add neatness to the campground. Most of the campsites are on the outside of the loop, with one pump well and two sets of vault toilets for each of the two loops.

The second loop is much like the first, except it has more vertical variation and meanders a bit. There are also several double campsites for larger groups or families. Most of the campsites are very appealing and don't have the beaten-down look of some heavily used campgrounds. This second loop is more popular, though it's hard to figure out why. The campground as a whole is large but doesn't seem crowded; rather, it feels forgotten.

And the scenery is as appealing as anywhere in the national forest. Take a look around on the Bishop Knob Loop Trail, which makes a 2-mile circuit of the campground. Start your walk near the campground pay station toward Forest Service Road 101, and turn right at a trail sign. Walk the serene woods to intersect the Cranberry Ridge Trail and turn right again, following the Cranberry Ridge Trail for a distance back to the loop trail. Turn right again; then pass over the dam of a pond just before returning to the campground.

Further trekking on the Cranberry Ridge Trail away from the loop hike will take you 3 miles to a pretty pond on the upper stretch of Glade Run. On the drive into the campground, near the turn onto FR 101, you passed the fenced Black Cherry Seed Orchard. The Forest Service is breeding a

:: Ratings

BEAUTY: ★ ★ ★
PRIVACY: ★ ★ ★ ★
SPACIOUSNESS: ★ ★ ★
QUIET: ★ ★ ★ ★ ★
SECURITY: ★ ★ ★
CLEANLINESS: ★ ★ ★ ★

:: Key Information

ADDRESS: Bishop Knob, Box 110, Richwood, WV 26261	**FACILITIES:** Pump well, vault toilets
OPERATED BY: U.S. Forest Service	**PARKING:** At campsites only
CONTACT: 304-846-2695, www.fs.usda.gov/mnf	**FEE:** $8 per night
	ELEVATION: 3,100 feet
OPEN: April–November	
SITES: 55	**RESTRICTIONS:**
SITE AMENITIES: Picnic table, fire grate, lantern post	■ **Pets:** On leash only
ASSIGNMENT: First come, first served; no reservations	■ **Fires:** In fire grates only
	■ **Alcohol:** At campsites only
REGISTRATION: Self-registration on-site	■ **Vehicles:** None
	■ **Other:** 14-day stay limit

superior strain of black cherry trees here for planting in other areas of the forest. The Adkins Rockhouse Trail starts near the orchard. You can take the Adkins Rockhouse Trail 2 miles down to the Gauley River and some good swimming holes.

The Williams and Cranberry rivers are also just a few miles away by car. Along these watercourses are quality trout fishing, but even if you don't catch one, you will have had an eyeful of pretty riverine sights. If you want a view from on high, head over to Red Oak Knob, where a fire tower stands at 3,707

feet. Drive just a short distance down FR 101 from the campground to FR 82, which may or may not be gated. If you do have to walk, the 3-mile trek from the gate is more than worth the effort.

The trip to Red Oak Knob fire tower also makes a great bike ride from Bishop Knob. Sometimes the fire tower is open, but if not, you can still climb the steps to just below the observation room for a good look over the Cranberry and Williams river valleys. Either way, your $8 investment will have paid off in scenic dividends.

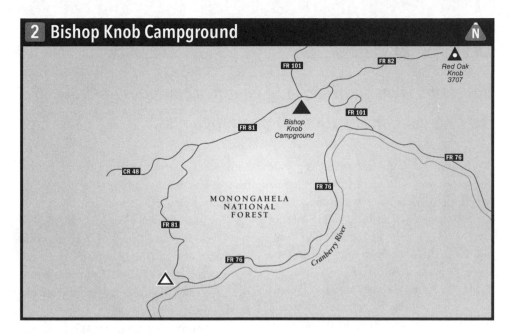

2 Bishop Knob Campground

:: Getting There

From Richwood, drive east on WV 39/55 for 0.5 mile to Cranberry Road (FR 76). Turn left on Cranberry Road and follow it nearly 3 miles to a signed intersection. FR 76 veers left and is the only gravel road at this intersection. Follow FR 76 for 4 miles to FR 81. Turn left on FR 81 and follow it 6 miles to FR 101. Turn right on FR 101 and follow it 0.1 mile to Bishop Knob Campground, which will be on your right.

GPS COORDINATES   N38° 20.319'   W80° 29.333'

3

Blue Bend

Blue Bend is an old-time, old-fashioned campground built by the Civilian Conservation Corps in the 1930s.

Blue Bend is named for a deep blue swimming hole in Anthony Creek, which flows right past the campground. This was probably a favorite cooling-off spot long before the Civilian Conservation Corps developed this campground during the Great Depression; it is still a great place to swim. Blue Bend Campground has evolved into a place where campers return time and again to pitch their tents under the tall hemlock forest. The forest service has a great system of trails in the immediate area, as well as forest drives leading to attractive sights in the vicinity.

Pass the pay station and drop into a forest of evergreens on a gravel road. Rhododendron forms the primary understory, making for good campsite privacy. On your left is the first restroom facility. There are campsites on both sides of the road. Anthony Creek flows off in the distance, with eight campsites lined up along the creek.

The CCC did a good job of spreading out the sites. Wood borders delineate the camping areas. White pine, tulip poplar, and maple complement the abundance of hemlock. Some of the campsites are set far from the road, so you have to walk a bit to get to your picnic table and fire ring. These sites are generally the most private.

Come to a small turnaround loop with more hardwoods. Three campsites spoke off the turnaround. Two are directly streamside. These are the most coveted campsites at Blue Bend.

The number of campsites at Blue Bend, 22, is almost ideal. It's large enough that all the sites aren't constantly taken, but it's not so big you feel like you are in a tent suburb. Apart from the summer holidays, you should be able to get a campsite at 6 p.m. on Friday, if not at noon on a Saturday, during high summer. Reserving a campsite can eliminate the worry and doubt. You'll have no trouble finding a campsite during the shoulder seasons or winter. In fact, September would be a good time to come. The crowds are mostly gone, but the creek is still warm enough to swim. And creek swimming is the best.

The CCC built stone patio beaches on either side of Blue Bend. These spots are good for relaxing streamside. You can access the far side of Blue Bend via a wooden swinging bridge. The patio on this side of the bridge has woods grown up all around. It is fun, however, to cross over the bridge and swim across to the main patio beach.

Anthony Creek is good for trout and smallmouth bass fishing. The waterway is

:: Ratings

BEAUTY: ★ ★ ★ ★
PRIVACY: ★ ★ ★ ★
SPACIOUSNESS: ★ ★ ★ ★
QUIET: ★ ★ ★ ★
SECURITY: ★ ★ ★ ★
CLEANLINESS: ★ ★ ★ ★

:: Key Information

ADDRESS: Blue Bend, 410 E. Main St., White Sulphur Springs, WV 24986

OPERATED BY: U.S. Forest Service

CONTACT: 304-536-2144, **www.fs.usda .gov/mnf;** reservations 877-444-6777, **reserveamerica.com**

OPEN: March–November

SITES: 22

SITE AMENITIES: Picnic table, fire ring, lantern post

ASSIGNMENT: First come, first served unless reserved

REGISTRATION: Self-registration on-site

FACILITIES: Warm showers, flush toilets, water

PARKING: At campsites only

FEE: $10 per night

ELEVATION: 1,950 feet

RESTRICTIONS:
- **Pets:** On leash only
- **Fires:** In fire rings only
- **Alcohol:** At campsites only
- **Vehicles:** None
- **Other:** 14-day stay limit

stocked regularly with trout during spring. Anthony Creek flows into the Greenbrier River, which is a noted smallmouth bass fishery. The Greenbrier is also known for the 75-mile Greenbrier River Trail. I have pedaled this path in its entirety and pronounce it a fine Mountain State adventure, no matter how many or few miles you pedal on this rail trail.

Blue Bend has its own set of trails. The Blue Bend Loop Trail is 5 miles long, enough to justify a good, long dip in Anthony Creek after you complete the hike. Cross the swinging bridge, and head downstream until you come to the Anthony Creek Trail at mile 1.6. Turn left and climb up the side of Round Mountain, reaching a backpacking shelter at 2.7 miles. Cross over Round Mountain and drop back down to Anthony Creek, passing some overlooks facing north. Cross back over the swinging bridge to end your loop.

Anglers will want to continue down the Anthony Creek Trail from its junction

with the Blue Bend Loop Trail. The Anthony Creek Trail parallels the stream for 3 more miles to the South Boundary Trail. You can continue on the Anthony Creek Trail to the Greenbrier River, but it necessitates a ford of Anthony Creek. Most hikers will return 4.6 miles to the campground. Hard-core hikers can head up the South Boundary Trail for 5 miles to Big Draft Road, then 3.5 miles on Big Draft Road, then another 1.1 miles back to Blue Bend for a blistering 14-miler.

You may want to consider touring by car instead. Just across from the campground entrance is Forest Service Road 139. It leads 3.5 miles up to Hopkins Lookout at 3,294 feet. Here, you can get mountaintop vistas of Little Creek Valley without all the effort. Or you can go left out of the campground and follow Anthony Creek Road 4 miles to the Gunpowder Overlook. Below is the Greenbrier River and Anthony Creek Gorge. Around Blue Bend, it seems everywhere you look there is attractive mountain scenery.

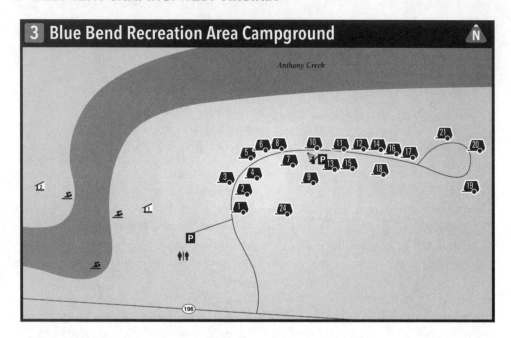

:: Getting There

From White Sulphur Springs, travel north on WV 92 for 9 miles to CR 16 (Little Creek Road). Turn left on CR 16 and follow it 2 miles to CR 16/2 (Blue Bend Road). Continue on CR 16/2 and come to Blue Bend Campground on your left in 2 more miles.

GPS COORDINATES   N37° 55.300′   W80° 16.102′

4

Cranberry

This campground is the gateway to the Cranberry Backcountry—haven for hikers, bikers, and anglers.

Cranberry Campground lies in a valley at the confluence of Mill Branch and the Cranberry River. This flat was once settled and farmed by early pioneers before West Virginia was a state. The area retains some pastoral character yet is surrounded by wild wooded mountains. Just a walk away is the Cranberry Backcountry, a good setting for hiking, biking, and fishing. When you're done exploring the Cranberry Backcountry, you can return to this quiet little valley campground. And if you're lucky, you'll return to one of the two walk-in tent sites, or any other campsite, for that matter. Plan ahead, as Cranberry fills nearly every summer weekend.

As you follow the Cranberry River deep into the wooded mountains, suddenly the brightness of the partially open campground grabs your attention. Pass the fee station and pump well; then pull into the row of campsites to your right. These are situated in a pretty flat, broken by oaks, rhododendrons, and maples. Mown grassy areas and timbers add a landscaped, organized quality to the area. The campsites are

:: Ratings

BEAUTY: ★ ★ ★
PRIVACY: ★ ★ ★
SPACIOUSNESS: ★ ★ ★ ★
QUIET: ★ ★ ★
SECURITY: ★ ★ ★
CLEANLINESS: ★ ★ ★

large and well separated. Up on a hill to your left are the Cranberry Graves, which is the old cemetery of the early valley settlers. A couple more campsites lie at the end of the row just before it comes to the Cranberry Backcountry trailhead.

The main campground loop passes the fee station and a couple of campsites, then crosses often-dry Mill Branch on a bridge. The area here is much more open and sunny, with occasional trees on the inside of the loop. The outer part of the loop is heavily wooded. This is where the walk-in tent sites are. Park your car and walk across a small footbridge over Mill Branch. Come to two very shaded and secluded campsites along Mill Branch that are the best in tent camping here. They have the normal campsite amenities, plus distance from the road.

Other campsites lie back on the main loop. These are very large and offer a wide array of sun and shade punctuated with brush along Mill Branch, which bisects the loop. The campsites get larger as the loop swings around toward the Cranberry River. The sites are usually occupied by pop-ups and bigger rigs. Don't camp here.

However, after finding a good site, explore the Cranberry Backcountry. Your main avenue of exploration is gated Forest Service Road 76. It parallels the Cranberry River beyond the campground and goes for 16 miles all the way to the Cranberry Glades Botanical Area. No private cars are allowed.

:: Key Information

ADDRESS: Cranberry, Box 110, Richwood, WV 26261	**FACILITIES:** Pump well, vault toilets
OPERATED BY: U.S. Forest Service	**PARKING:** At campsites and at tent camping area
CONTACT: 304-846-2695, www.fs.usda.gov/mnf	**FEE:** $10 per night
OPEN: Mid-May–November	**ELEVATION:** 2,500 feet
SITES: 30	**RESTRICTIONS:**
SITE AMENITIES: Picnic table, fire grate, lantern post	■ **Pets:** On leash only
ASSIGNMENT: First come, first served; no reservations	■ **Fires:** In fire grates only
	■ **Alcohol:** At campsites only
REGISTRATION: Self-registration on-site	■ **Vehicles:** None
	■ **Other:** 14-day stay limit

Technically, the road changes to FR 102, but aesthetically it only gets prettier as you head upriver. Along the way are trail shelters and numerous hiking and fishing opportunities. Anglers will be pleased to know the 50-foot-wide Cranberry River is stocked with legal-catch-size trout January–May and twice in autumn. Fishing can be good on the roadside sections of the Cranberry River too.

Make a great 9-mile loop in the Cranberry Backcountry from the campground following FR 76 for 2 miles; then turn left on the Lick Branch Trail (Forest Trail 212). Begin to look for signs of an old lumber camp as the trail climbs alongside many small falls for 2 miles to the North–South Trail (Forest Trail 688). Turn left and follow the North–South Trail along the ridge until it drops off the mountainside and returns to the Cranberry River and the campground.

Bicyclers take note: The Cranberry Backcountry has many wilderness qualities, yet it is not a designated wilderness, which means you can enjoy the trails of the Cranberry Backcountry as well. FR 76 makes a great road for pedaling, but don't wreck while enjoying that tumbling riverside scenery. The side trails aren't as biker friendly, but there is another gated road paralleling Dogway Fork (FR 78) that adds enough mileage to exhaust you. FR 78 spurs off FR 76 at 6 miles. Get a forest map and go have a ball!

4 Cranberry Campground

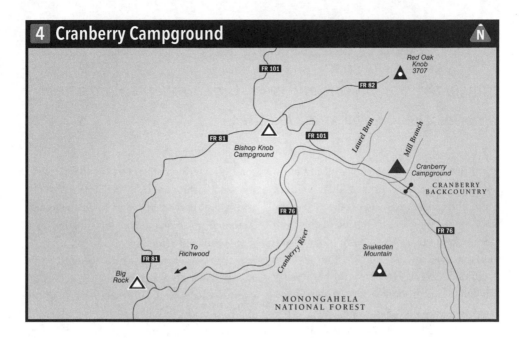

:: Getting There

From Richwood, drive east on WV 39/55 for 0.5 mile to Cranberry Road (FR 76). Turn left on Cranberry Road, and follow it nearly 3 miles to an intersection. FR 76 veers left and is the only gravel road at this intersection. Follow FR 76 for 9 miles to Cranberry Campground, which will be on your left just before the road dead-ends.

GPS COORDINATES   N38° 19.467'   W80° 26.467'

5

Day Run

Stay in this quiet locale and enjoy the Cranberry Wilderness, among other nearby forest features.

The major attraction at Day Run Campground is the upper Williams River. Here, you can fish for trout or take a dip in the cool mountain waters. Outside of that, you have to get in a vehicle to reach other attractions, such as the Cranberry Wilderness, the Highland Scenic Highway, the Cranberry Visitor Center, the view from High Rocks, the Cranberry Glades, and the Falls of Hills Creek. Day Run, a small, secluded campground, allows access to all these attractions yet has that slow-moving, old-time national forest campground ambience.

Day Run is situated in a flat alongside Williams River. I'd bet this flat was once settled. It's too level and too open not to have been a farm long ago. Even so, Day Run is an old campground. Rocks and posts delineate the campsites, which support an interesting array of vegetation. Hawthorn, buckeye, sumac, crab apple, and ash grow between the grass and brush areas. Pass the fee station on a gravel road, and campsite 1 is on your left, beneath some trees next to a grassy area by the pump well. Across the gravel road, you'll find campsite 2 in a deep, riverine woodland alongside Williams River. On your right, pass vault toilets for each gender. Across from this is campsite 3, shaded by a large crab apple tree.

Trees and brush conspire to keep campers' privacy at a maximum, especially at campsites 4, 5, and 6. Campsite 5 is possibly the best of this bunch—a large area located near the river. Campsite 7 is also by the river but more out in the open.

A turnaround loop begins past campsite 7. Along the loop are more examples of sun and shade mixtures to suit most any tent camper. I stayed at campsite 9, mostly sunny yet nicely shaded by a huge crab apple tree. I'd been rained on the night before and dried my gear in the sun while relaxing beneath the old crab apple. This site has a footpath leading to the Williams River, as do other riverside campsites here. The last three sites offer more varieties of sun and shade, plus a whole lot of privacy. Near campsite 12 is another set of vault toilets.

The small size of this campground makes for a serene setting, and the less developed, rustic nature of Day Run deters most big rigs. Enjoy this campground almost any weekend, except during summer holidays.

To find the right roads and trails, get a Monongahela National Forest map before you come to Day Run. There are many attractions here, but they are spread out. Your first trip should be to the Cranberry

:: Ratings

BEAUTY: ★ ★ ★ ★
PRIVACY: ★ ★ ★ ★ ★
SPACIOUSNESS: ★ ★ ★ ★ ★
QUIET: ★ ★ ★ ★
SECURITY: ★ ★ ★
CLEANLINESS: ★ ★ ★

:: Key Information

ADDRESS: Day Run Campground, P.O. Box 210, Marlinton, WV 24954

OPERATED BY: U.S. Forest Service

CONTACT: 304-799-4334, www.fs.usda.gov/mnf

OPEN: April 1–November

SITES: 12

SITE AMENITIES: Picnic table, fire grate, lantern post, waste can

ASSIGNMENT: First come, first served; no reservations

REGISTRATION: Self-registration on-site

FACILITIES: Pump well, vault toilets

PARKING: At campsites only

FEE: $8 per night

ELEVATION: 3,100 feet

RESTRICTIONS:
- **Pets:** On leash only
- **Fire:** In fire grates only
- **Alcohol:** At campsites only
- **Vehicles:** None
- **Other:** 14-day stay limit

Visitor Center. Check out the interpretive displays, and figure out what is most appealing. A drive on the Highland Scenic Highway is a sure thing. Stop at some of the numerous overlooks to gaze at the mountains and valleys below. There are also trails that will reward you with even more spectacular views. The Black Mountain Trail makes a 4.6-mile loop through the high country. Or try the High Rocks Trail for a truly first-rate view. It takes you on a 3.2-mile out-and-back hike that looks east toward old Virginia.

Several other trails spur off Highland Scenic Highway into the Cranberry Wilderness. The Forks of the Cranberry Trail leads 2.1 miles to a rocky vista. Check out the Cranberry Glades for a look at a tundra environment, unique this far south. A half-mile boardwalk traverses the open bogs of the glades. For a water experience, go to the Falls of Hills Creek Scenic Area. Here, a trail traces three picturesque waterfalls along Hills Creek. This walk is especially dramatic after a rain and is sure to return you to your campground on Williams River feeling fulfilled.

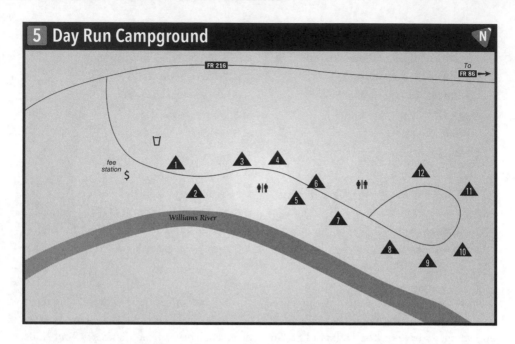

:: Getting There

From Marlinton, drive north on US 210 for 7 miles to Highland Scenic Highway. Turn left on Highland Scenic Highway and follow it south for 10 miles to FR 86. Head south on FR 86 for 3 miles to FR 216. Turn right on FR 216 and follow it 1 mile to Day Run Campground, which will be on your left.

GPS COORDINATES   N38° 17.183′   W80° 13.001′

6

Horseshoe

The primary camping area is nice, but the tent campers' area is even better.

This is the kind of well-landscaped campground that makes the most of its natural setting and makes other campgrounds look bad. The campground is open but not too sunny. The campsites are neat but not overdone. Horseshoe Run sings its way downstream, while the mountainside across the campground rises high above Horseshoe Run. Wood smoke curls through the large white pines.

Once there was a 13-site loop and a picnic area at Horseshoe. The original loop itself was worthy of making this book, but then the old picnic area was turned into a walk-in tent campers' camp. The creekside setting is near ideal for tent campers—plenty of privacy yet convenient to campground amenities and your car. The tent campers' area made Horseshoe Campground even better and is a must for anyone tent camping in the upper Cheat River area.

This is an all-inclusive recreation area that should keep you entertained, that is, if you enjoy mountain streams, hiking trails, and canoe trips.

:: Ratings

BEAUTY: ★ ★ ★ ★ ★
PRIVACY: ★ ★ ★
SPACIOUSNESS: ★ ★ ★ ★
QUIET: ★ ★ ★
SECURITY: ★ ★ ★ ★
CLEANLINESS: ★ ★ ★ ★

The entrance road drops down to flat land alongside Horseshoe Run. The neatness of the campground is immediately evident. An open, grassy area lies in the center of the main loop, which is ringed by towering white pines. Smaller trees, such as yellow birch, and some rhododendron provide an understory. A lower wooded flat lies between the campground and Horseshoe Run. The campsites begin just past the pay station. A campground host is there for the well-being of all campers, and elevated tent pads filled with small gravel mean dry sleeping even when it's raining.

The campground is twice the size it could be for so few sites. Most any combination of sun and shade is there for the taking. Most sites are first come, first served, but eight electric sites are available for reservation. A pair of modern vault toilets is stationed between campsites 8 and 9. A footbridge crosses McKinley Run into a large field next to the campground. Kids run and play on the grass. Older kids throw Frisbees. Others lie in the sun by the creek. The final sites continue along McKinley Run, and the loop ends.

Turn left and drive to the tent campers' parking area to get to the best in tent camping at Horseshoe—and some of the best in West Virginia. Leave your car parked by the big field, and enter a much more wooded and less groomed (read: natural) area than the main campground. White pine, birch, and

:: Key Information

ADDRESS: Horseshoe, P.O. Box 368, Parsons, WV 26287	**REGISTRATION:** By phone, online, or self-registration on-site
OPERATED BY: U.S. Forest Service	**FACILITIES:** Water spigots, vault toilets
CONTACT: 304-478-3251, **www.fs.usda.gov/mnf;** reservations 877-444-6777, **reserveamerica.com**	**PARKING:** At campsites only for Main Loop or tent campers' parking area
OPEN: May 5–November 31	**FEE:** $20 per night electric sites, $15 others
SITES: 21	**ELEVATION:** 1,750 feet
SITE AMENITIES: Main Loop: electricity, picnic table, fire grate, tent pad, lantern post; Tent Camper's Area: picnic table, grill, fire grate	**RESTRICTIONS:**
	■ **Pets:** On leash only
	■ **Fires:** In fire grates only
ASSIGNMENT: Reservations accepted but not required	■ **Alcohol:** At campsites only
	■ **Vehicles:** None

an understory of evergreen are your campsite borders. These walk-in sites ensure an RV-free zone. Follow a path that leads past two campsites under tall trees next to a hill. Most of the remaining tent campsites lie along Horseshoe Run in one good setting after another. Between the tent campers' area and the big field are the bathrooms for tent campers. Water spigots are located here and in the main campground.

By now, you have noticed Horseshoe Run. There is a nice swimming hole by the field that's great for cooling off. Trout fishermen will want to get a little bit away from the swimming hole to vie for trout. If you want to try another watery experience, canoe the Cheat River, where the bass fishing is said to be good. Nearby Blackwater Outdoor Adventures will provide canoes and a shuttle (for a fee) on a 35-mile stretch of river that's perfect for paddling. Pick the length of your trip. You can contact them at 304-478-3775 or **blackwateroutdoors.com.**

Trails leave the campground if you want to hike. The Two Camp Trail (Forest Trail 111) leaves the campground near the pay station. It heads downstream for a level 0.4 mile before intersecting the Losh Trail (Forest Trail 155). Take the Losh Trail across Horseshoe Run on a footbridge to climb 1.8 miles to a trail shelter in the high country. Turn on the Dorman Ridge Trail (Forest Trail 153) for a ramble through open areas with mountain panoramas. Return the way you came.

Up McKinley Run, the side stream by the main campground, is another footpath (Forest Trail 154) that climbs along its namesake stream toward Close Mountain. If you want to see some waterfalls, try the Maxwell Run Trail (Forest Trail 157). It starts about a mile back down the road toward Parsons and climbs 2 miles up Maxwell Run in a narrow valley. Return the way you came. After you've experienced Horseshoe Campground, odds are you will return.

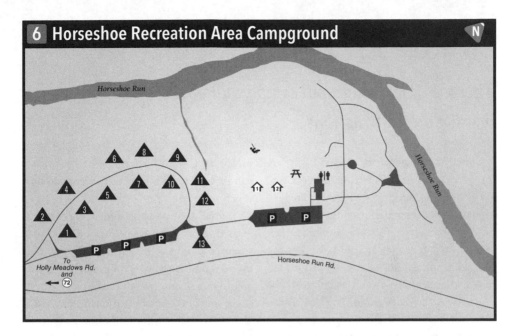

6 Horseshoe Recreation Area Campground

:: Getting There

From Parsons, drive north on WV 72 for 6 miles to the Cheat River Bridge at St. George. There is a sign for Horseshoe Campground here. Cross the Cheat River and enter St. George. Soon turn right on Holly Meadows Road (CR 1) and follow it for 3 miles to Horseshoe Run Road (CR 7). Turn left on Horseshoe Run Road and follow it for 3.3 miles to Horseshoe Campground, which will be on your left.

GPS COORDINATES   N39° 10.688′   W79° 36.103′

7

Island

This old-time, traditional campground boasts a variety of nearby forest attractions.

Island Campground, located on an island of the East Fork Greenbrier River, is small, rustic, and free. Hikers and anglers enjoy the little-used gem of the East Fork Trail, which starts at the campground. Other nearby natural attractions are Lake Buffalo, also with hiking and fishing opportunities, and Gaudineer Scenic Area, which features an old-growth spruce stand. The Civil War–era Cheat Summit Fort also merits a visit.

Pull off WV 28 and travel the gravel road to Island Campground. You will first notice the vault toilets off to your right. This is also the beginning of the East Fork Trail. Immediately to your left is a gravel road leading 50 yards to an isolated campsite in a stand of evergreens that offers maximum privacy, even though it is the closest to WV 28. Traffic can barely be heard over the babbling of the East Fork Greenbrier River.

Continue forward and cross a wood bridge over a small streamlet. To your left lies a somewhat shaded campsite beside the watercourse. This site is on the small side but has no other campsites nearby. Cross a second little wood bridge over another wet

meander. To your left is another streamside campsite. This site has adequate size and much privacy.

Finally, come to a vehicle turnaround with three campsites spoking off. The first site on the right is the largest. It is encircled by trees and fairly near the East Fork. Next, an old road runs straight to the creek where there was once a bridge. An excellent, well-shaded tent area hunkers beside this, down in a flat. Trees crowd the sky overhead, and the East Fork is just a few steps away. Here, tent campers will be sung to sleep by the stream.

The final campsite is level and well shaded, if short on room. Since the campground only has a few sites, most folks pass Island Campground by for the bigger, more publicized area campgrounds. However, it has been a traditional camping ground for decades and will fill only on summer holidays and a few great-weather weekends.

Island Campground makes a fine base camp for exploring the East Fork Greenbrier Valley. The East Fork Trail runs along this stream and is a pleasure in any season. Spring brings wildflowers aplenty. In summer, anglers fish for trout or cool off in swimming holes. Fall's paintbrush warms the valley with vibrant colors, and in winter the lack of mandatory fords makes this a viable hike. However, take care during higher flows.

Lake Buffalo, which you passed on the way to Island from Bartow, is 20 acres of aquatic beauty. The clear water, set in a

:: Ratings

BEAUTY: ★ ★ ★
PRIVACY: ★ ★ ★ ★
SPACIOUSNESS: ★ ★ ★ ★
QUIET: ★ ★ ★
SECURITY: ★ ★ ★
CLEANLINESS: ★ ★ ★

:: Key Information

ADDRESS: Island Campground, Box 67, Bartow, WV 24920	**REGISTRATION:** None
	FACILITIES: Vault toilets; bring water
OPERATED BY: U.S. Forest Service	**PARKING:** At campsites only
CONTACT: 304-456-3335, www.fs.usda.gov/mnf	**FEE:** None
	ELEVATION: 2,600 feet
OPEN: Mid-April–November	
SITES: 6	**RESTRICTIONS:**
	■ **Pets:** On leash only
SITE AMENITIES: Picnic table, fire grate, lantern post	■ **Fires:** In fire grates only
	■ **Alcohol:** At campsites only
ASSIGNMENT: First come, first served; no reservations	■ **Vehicles:** None
	■ **Other:** 14-day stay limit

mountain valley, offers fishing for trout, bass, and bream. Anglers and hikers commonly use the trail around the lake.

On US 250 beyond Bartow is the Gaudineer Scenic Area, where 140 acres of forestland have been set aside for their exceptional beauty. Fifty of these acres are completely virgin woods—primarily red spruce, some of which exceed 3 feet in diameter and are more than 300 years old. You'll also find yellow birch, beech, and maple.

A short distance beyond Gaudineer Scenic Area lies Cheat Summit Fort. This Union Fort was built in 1861 to protect the Staunton-Parkersburg Turnpike. Confederates and Yankees skirmished in the region. This was allegedly the site where the telegraph was first used during the Civil War. There are good views from the ridge, and you will find Fort Milroy Cemetery nearby. Also nearby is Strip Mine Trail, which offers more views and insight into West Virginia stripmining culture. To get to this area, turn left from US 250 near Cheat Bridge, turn right at the T junction, and go 1 mile to the top of the ridge.

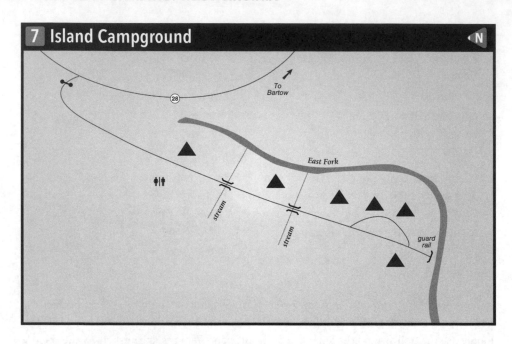

:: Getting There

From Bartow, at the intersection of US 250 and WV 28/92, head north on WV 28/ US 250 for 2.2 miles. As US 250 veers right, continue on WV 28 for 2.6 miles. Island Campground will be on your left.

GPS COORDINATES   N38° 34.761'   W79° 42.284'

8

Kumbrabow State Forest

This is one of the state's most underutilized natural resources.

This forest is in the high country. In fact, it is West Virginia's highest state forest, with elevations ranging from 3,000 to 3,855 feet. Its forest is northern hardwoods: cherry and yellow birch. Before the state acquired Kumbrabow, the mountains here were logged for the immense stands of spruce and hemlock. The forest has since recovered to become one of the most attractive, least used forests in the entire state. I surmise that limited access and lack of knowledge lead to the absence of campers. But now you have no excuse not to have a great tent-camping experience here.

Mill Creek Campground is set alongside Mill Creek, which native brook trout call home. Mill Creek is off to your left, with a smaller creek coming in to your right. Descend among rhododendron, passing a water pump. Notice that the first seven campsites have stone fireplaces in addition to the fire grates. These are leftovers from the handiwork of the Civilian Conservation Corps, who built this original camping area. The sites are medium to small but very scenic, especially if you like camping on a tumbling stream.

:: Ratings

BEAUTY: ★ ★ ★ ★
PRIVACY: ★ ★ ★
SPACIOUSNESS: ★ ★ ★
QUIET: ★ ★ ★ ★ ★
SECURITY: ★ ★ ★ ★ ★
CLEANLINESS: ★ ★ ★ ★

Cross a low-water bridge over Mill Creek and come to the "newer" camping area. A short road to your left leads to two streamside campsites. The main road passes between a field and the stream. These streamside campsites are larger, with rhododendron and large stones providing campsite barriers. Pass a disabled-accessible campsite and a second water pump. A few more campsites are strung along Mill Creek. I would stay at any of these campsites; they are all good. Bring your change—the state forest has installed coin-operated showers and a laundry at the forest headquarters. You can get a campsite here anytime, barring summer holidays. Be apprised that the shoulder seasons can be chilly. Snow can fall in April, and generally any night will be cool—perfect for that evening campfire—at this extremely rural, rustic getaway that is like a trip back in time.

The forest covers 9,474 acres of rugged mountain land, where the bears roam and the native trout swim free. The primary attraction of Kumbrabow is angling for the native brookies along Mill Creek and its tributaries. Tributaries, such as Meatbox Run and Potato Hole Run, are not as productive as Mill Creek but provide the angler with a scenic experience, even if the fish aren't biting.

If you like hiking in solitude, come here. Chances are, you won't see another person, but you may see some wildlife. The Rich Mountain Fire Trail follows the northern border of the forest and takes you to

:: Key Information

ADDRESS: Kumbrabow State Forest, Box 65, Huttonsville, WV 26273	**FACILITIES:** Vault toilet, pump well, coin-operated shower, and laundry at forest headquarters
OPERATED BY: West Virginia State Parks	
CONTACT: 304-335-2219, **kumbrabow.com**	**PARKING:** At campsites only
	FEE: $14 per night
OPEN: Mid-April–mid-December	**ELEVATION:** 3,000 feet
SITES: 13	
SITE AMENITIES: Picnic table, fire grate	**RESTRICTIONS:**
ASSIGNMENT: First come, first served; no reservations	■ **Pets:** On leash only
	■ **Fires:** In fire grates only
	■ **Alcohol:** Prohibited
REGISTRATION: At park office or ranger will come by to register you	■ **Vehicles:** None
	■ **Other:** 14-day stay limit

the highest point in the area, Buck Knob. Several connector paths drop off from Rich Mountain. The Raven Rocks Trail drops sharply from the Rich Mountain Fire Trail to a rock overlook. You can use the Potato Hole Run and Meatbox Run trails for a loop.

From the campground, follow the Mill Creek Trail down past the forest cabins, and come to Mill Creek Falls. This path can also be used for fishing access. The Mill Ridge trails are on the far side of Mill Creek. There are loop opportunities here, using the Mill Ridge, Clay Run, and Mowery paths.

Also on forest grounds is the old Camp Bowers. This is an old CCC camp that was occupied from 1934 to 1941. You can see remains of where the young men lived while developing Kumbrabow. By the way, Kumbrabow is not an American Indian name. It is the agglomeration of three names of families: Kump, Brady, and Bowers, who helped in the acquisition of the forestland.

A nearby attraction is the hamlet of Helvetia. It is a community of Swiss descendants who originally settled there in the 1860s. They have preserved many Swiss traditions. There is a historic district in the town. To get there, pass the forest office, turn right on Turkeybone Road (County Road 45), and make a scenic drive to Helvetia. The Swiss were right to settle in this high, mountainous section of West Virginia.

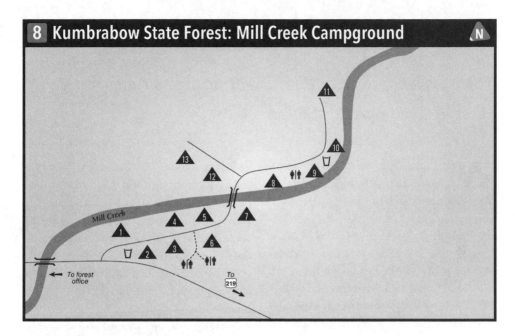

:: Getting There

From Huttonsville, drive south on US 219 for 7 miles to Kumbrabow Road (CR 216).
There will be a sign for the state forest here. Turn right on CR 216 and follow the
gravel road 5 miles into the state forest.

GPS COORDINATES   N38° 39.386'   W80° 04.284'

9

Lake Sherwood

There is plenty to do at this recreation area situated on West Virginia's prettiest lake.

West Virginia has many pretty valleys bordered by high mountains. That describes much of the state. However, you just might agree with me that the valley of Meadow Creek, bordered by Meadow Creek Mountain on one side and the state-line range of the Alleghenies on the other, may be the Mountain State's prettiest valley. Meadow Creek was dammed in 1958, and Lake Sherwood was born. This capped off the scenery.

Lake Sherwood Recreation Area is very well kept. The developments did nothing to spoil the natural allure. Swimming, fishing, hiking, and all-around relaxing are on the agenda when you find yourself at the terminus of Lake Sherwood Road.

As you drive up, Lake Sherwood will be on your right. The swim beaches and main boat landing are over that way too. Then come to the year-round camping area, West Shore Loop. The forest is dominated by white pine, oak, and hickory, with a lot of dogwood. Wooden posts delineate the campsites. Several campsites overlook the lake from a bluff. This loop has a full bathhouse for summer and vault toilets and pump well for the off-season. The sites are very spacious, which adds to the privacy. Some campers pull their boats right up to the shore from the lake.

The Pine Run Loop is on a little higher and drier land. It is heavier on Virginia pine and has a more open forest but is still very pretty. The main loop here swings out toward the lake and has several sites that overlook the reservoir. There is another spur road on the far side of a rill that has very large campsites that can be reserved. At the end of this road is another boat launch.

The final loop, Meadow Creek, is also in a pine-oak-hickory complex. All 35 sites can be reserved here. The campsites are so well designed, well spaced, and big that they attract some RVs. Just grin and bear it here; this place is worth it. The spur road with another boat launch has some campsites very close to the lake. The loop turns away from the lake, climbs a hill, and splits. There are more good campsites on both roads.

All the loops have campground hosts who are making their contribution, giving Lake Sherwood that well-cared-for look. Water spigots are spread through all the loops, as are bathhouses. If you are coming from far away, reserve a campsite. Lake Sherwood deservedly fills on all major holidays and many weekends and stays busy during the week in high summer. Autumn is an

:: Ratings

BEAUTY: ★ ★ ★ ★ ★
PRIVACY: ★ ★ ★ ★
SPACIOUSNESS: ★ ★ ★ ★
QUIET: ★ ★ ★ ★
SECURITY: ★ ★ ★ ★ ★
CLEANLINESS: ★ ★ ★ ★ ★

:: Key Information

ADDRESS: Lake Sherwood, 410 E. Main St., White Sulphur Springs, WV 24986

OPERATED BY: U.S. Forest Service

CONTACT: 304-536-2144, **www.fs.usda .gov/mnf;** reservations 877-444-6777, **reserveamerica.com**

OPEN: West Shore Loop: March–November; rest of campground: mid-May–early September

SITES: 95

SITE AMENITIES: Picnic table, fire grate, lantern post, tent pad

ASSIGNMENT: Reservations accepted but not required

REGISTRATION: Online, by phone, or at campground entrance kiosk

FACILITIES: Hot showers, flush toilets, water spigots

PARKING: At campsites only

FEE: $10–$16 single, $32 double per night

ELEVATION: 2,670 feet

RESTRICTIONS:

■ **Pets:** On leash only

■ **Fires:** In fire grates only

■ **Alcohol:** At campsites only

■ **Vehicles:** None

■ **Boats:** Electric motors only

■ **Other:** 14-day stay limit

excellent alternate time, with the fall colors reflecting off the lake.

The 144-acre impoundment lures anglers in for some potentially exciting fishing. Tiger muskie, large predatory fish, are stocked here. They can run 15 pounds or more. Largemouth bass, bluegill, and catfish round out the platter. Artificial fish-attracting reefs have been put in the lake. For the peace of all lake visitors, only electric motors are allowed.

Boats and canoes are available for rent near the main boat launch. Also near the launch are a bathhouse and two beaches. One beach is on the main shore; the other is on an island accessible by a wooden bridge. The swimming area is between the two beaches. You will rarely find a more attractive setting in which to cool off.

Several trails leave directly from the recreation area. The most notable is the Lake Sherwood Trail. It makes a 3.2-mile loop around the lake. This is a moderate walk suitable for the entire family. The Virginia Trail spurs off the Lake Sherwood Trail and heads 0.6 mile up to the Allegheny

Mountain Trail. From here, you walk the state-line ridge for 3.6 miles and gain views of Lake Sherwood and Lake Moomaw in Virginia.

The Meadow Creek Trail starts at the head of Lake Sherwood and parallels Meadow Creek, crossing the stream several times amid thickets of rhododendron, intersecting the Connector Trail at 2.7 miles. Here, you can turn right and make a 10-mile loop back to the Meadow Creek bridge at Lake Sherwood using the Allegheny Mountain and Lake Sherwood Trails. This is one of West Virginia's finest circuit hikes.

Bikers can pedal the recreation-area roads or head a mile up the Upper Meadow Trail to tackle the Meadow Creek Mountain. This old road runs along the crest of the ridge, offering scenic views into Lake Sherwood. You can continue north for 3-plus miles to intersect the Connector Trail for more loop possibilities. Another possibility is lying around your campsite taking in the scenery at West Virginia's prettiest lake. Come here and rate it for yourself.

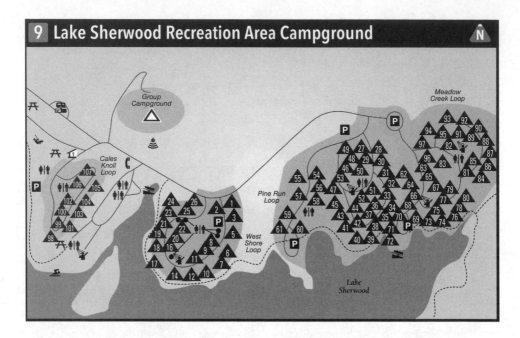

:: Getting There

From Exit 181 on I-64 at White Sulphur Springs, drive 15 miles north on WV 92 to Neola. From Neola, travel east on Lake Sherwood Road for 11 miles, and enter the recreation area.

GPS COORDINATES   N38° 00.470′   W80° 00.715′

10

Laurel Fork

Laurel Fork lies between two scenic wilderness areas.

This large, pretty, and free campground is situated between two of Monongahela National Forest's premier wilderness areas, Laurel Fork North and Laurel Fork South. Come here and plan to do a little exploring. And when you return to your campsite, you can enjoy ridgetop views and a relaxing place to contemplate the natural surroundings—a key element of tent camping.

Drop from Forest Service Road 14 into the Laurel Fork Valley. Come to a cleared area with forest buildings on your left. The forest service used this location as wildlife management headquarters, but the buildings are now unoccupied. Originally this was a Civilian Conservation Corps camp. You, however, can enjoy the area as a campground.

Turn right into the upper loop. This loop is huge for so few campsites. Attractive wood fences protect clear areas. Pass the pump well and come to a good campsite on your left, which lies between a row of Norway spruce trees and Laurel Fork. The loop splits right into a clearing dotted with a few trees. Three campsites are out in the open. They offer the maximum in spaciousness and have good views but no shade.

:: Ratings

BEAUTY: ★ ★ ★ ★
PRIVACY: ★ ★ ★
SPACIOUSNESS: ★ ★ ★ ★ ★
QUIET: ★ ★ ★ ★ ★
SECURITY: ★ ★ ★
CLEANLINESS: ★ ★ ★ ★

The fourth site is banked against the woods and has good views and afternoon shade. A pair of vault toilets is nearby, and beyond them is a great campsite beneath a grove of red pine. This shady site is adjacent to the Laurel River south trailhead. The loop swings around along Laurel Creek and passes two large sites that are directly on the creek and have good morning shade. There is also one open campsite in the center of the loop.

Return to the main road and cross Laurel Fork on a wood bridge. Immediately to your right is a lone, well-shaded, popular campsite that is along the river. Enter the lower loop, which is also oversized (as are the campsites). The center of the loop is grassy and has a covered picnic shelter. This large central clearing allows mountain views for all campers. More wood fences delineate the camping areas.

Pass a vault toilet on your right, and then come to the first campsite. It benefits from shady spruce and pine trees. This campsite is right next to the trail that enters the Laurel Fork North Wilderness. Just on the other side of the trailhead is a campsite that has good views and a mixture of sun and shade provided by spruce and hawthorn trees. Then there is a more open site right next to Laurel Fork that is coveted by campers. An open campsite by the water precedes a very large one that has it all: sun, shade, and river access.

The few campsites here may be the largest in all the state. The setting is very pretty,

:: Key Information

ADDRESS: Laurel Fork Campground, Box 67, Bartow, WV 24920

OPERATED BY: U.S. Forest Service

CONTACT: 304-456-3335, www.fs.usda.gov/mnf

OPEN: Year-round

SITES: 16

SITE AMENITIES: Picnic table, fire ring, lantern post, waste can

ASSIGNMENT: First come, first served; no reservations

REGISTRATION: None

FACILITIES: Vault toilet

PARKING: At campsites only

FEE: None

ELEVATION: 3,100 feet

RESTRICTIONS:

- **Pets:** On leash only
- **Fires:** In fire rings only
- **Alcohol:** At campsites only
- **Vehicles:** None
- **Other:** 14-day stay limit

but the price paid for the views is a lack of privacy. Expect Laurel Fork Campground to fill on summer holidays and some weekends. Try to come during the week in summer. A great time to visit is in autumn.

Campers here are of two stripes: those who like to explore, and those who like to relax. Active campers have two trails leaving right from the campground into the wilderness areas. Technically, they are both the Laurel River Trail, but one heads into Laurel Fork Wilderness North and the other into Laurel Fork Wilderness South. After you take a hike, you will understand why these scenic areas were protected as federally designated wilderness, totaling nearly 12,000 acres.

Take the Laurel River Trail from the upper loop, and head upstream along Laurel Fork, passing some attractive woods carpeted in ferns. Numerous meadows add to the scenery. Evidence of beavers is everywhere, and you may even see one of these industrious critters. A good destination is the confluence of Camp Five Run and Laurel Fork, 4 miles distant. Here is a large meadow and a shady evergreen thicket, where you can sprawl out in the sun or have a picnic in the shade. The Laurel River Trail also leaves the lower loop and passes many fields. The creek is bigger here and offers angling opportunities. It heads down several miles in an ever-widening valley. Be advised: These wilderness trails are not as well marked as most national forest paths.

I hiked both trails. As an active camper, I explored the wilderness areas, then joined the other Laurel Fork camper types, the relaxers, and stretched out on a hammock. It felt good to take in the scenery and enjoy another evening of tent camping in the Mountain State.

10 Laurel Fork Campground

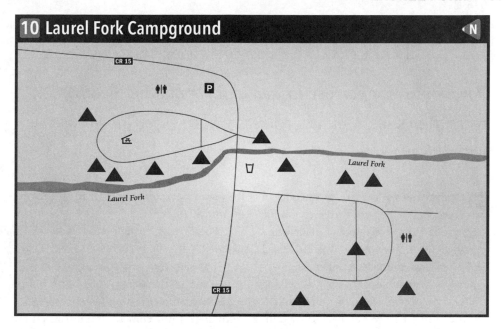

:: Getting There

From the post office in Glady, drive east on FR 422 for 4.6 miles to FR 14. Drive south on FR 14 for 0.3 mile to FR 423. Turn left on FR 423 and drive 1.5 miles down to Laurel Fork Campground.

GPS COORDINATES   N38° 44.421′   W79° 41.514′

11

Pocahontas

Pocahontas is often overlooked in favor of other nearby recreation sites. Mountain bikers will be especially pleased with this place.

Pocahontas is a great destination in many ways: It is an extremely scenic campground set in a forest of giant white pine beside a valley stream. It is little used and inexpensive and has quiet yet well-maintained mountain biking and hiking trails leaving directly from the campground. So why is it not more popular? The campground is a little too close to WV 92. The highway is not heavily traveled, but you can hear every car that passes by. If you can't overlook this fact, then read no further.

I was skeptical about Pocahontas myself, until I gave it a try. It was raining when I arrived, so I set up the tent, then fell asleep to the raindrops on the tent fly. Around 4 p.m. I awoke, and the rain had stopped, though the skies were still cloudy. After powering down some coffee, I took off up the Two Lick Run Trail, taking in the tranquil scenery. Later that night I sat beside the campfire, feeling sorry for all those passing by Pocahontas in their cars. By the way,

it was a Friday night and I had the campground all to myself.

Pocahontas Campground is set in a wooded flat along Cochran Creek. Leave WV 92, pass the Two Lick Run trailhead, and come to the pump well. Some pump wells have funny-tasting water, especially right after it first comes out, but this pump puts out nothing but pure, sweet water. And I've drunk a lot of pump-well water in my camping days. This is some of the finest I've ever had.

The first campsite is across from the pump well. You'll notice the forest overhead: there are huge white pines above an understory of maple, musclewood, hemlock, and a few oaks. Smaller trees thicken the understory. Then come to two more large campsites with a lot of privacy. Unfortunately, these are the closest to the road.

Swing around, and towering pines rise overhead. Large, isolated campsites are on the outside of the loop. Pass a small rill that meanders through the center of the loop. Now the oval parallels Cochran Creek. The forest is thicker, with more hemlock trees and some rhododendron. The last few sites border either Cochran Creek or the small campground rill. Two vault toilets, one for each gender, complete the campground.

I believe you can get a campsite here just about any day it is open. I am all for leaving the sounds of civilization behind,

:: Ratings

> BEAUTY: ★ ★ ★ ★ ★
> PRIVACY: ★ ★ ★
> SPACIOUSNESS: ★ ★ ★ ★
> QUIET: ★ ★ ★
> SECURITY: ★ ★ ★
> CLEANLINESS: ★ ★ ★ ★

:: Key Information

ADDRESS: Pocahontas, P.O. Box 210, Marlinton, WV 24954-0210

OPERATED BY: U.S. Forest Service

CONTACT: 304-799-4334, **www.fs.usda.gov/mnf**

OPEN: April–November

SITES: 8

SITE AMENITIES: Picnic table, fire grate, lantern post

ASSIGNMENT: First come, first served; no reservations

REGISTRATION: Self-registration on-site

FACILITIES: Pump well, vault toilets

PARKING: At campsites only

FEE: $8 per night

ELEVATION: 2,490 feet

RESTRICTIONS:
- **Pets:** On leash only
- **Fires:** In fire grates only
- **Alcohol:** At campsites only
- **Vehicles:** None
- **Other:** 14-day stay limit

but the advantages of Pocahontas simply outweigh the disadvantages. It seemed I had my own private recreation area. No one was on the trails, hiking or biking. And this was in mid-May.

Mountain bikers especially shouldn't miss Pocahontas. Two loops marked for the pedaling set leave directly from the campground. The Middle Mountain Route leaves the campground and goes left on WV 92 to Forest Service Road 790. Climb FR 790, a gated road, to FR 962. Travel 6 miles north to the Middle Mountain Trail for some single-track action, then on down to WV 39, then right again on WV 92 for a 13-mile loop. The Lockridge Mountain Route is a little easier. Turn right out of the campground on WV 92, then right on WV 39 for 0.5 mile. Turn left on FR 55, and then start your return on the gated FR 345 and circle back via Rimel Picnic Area. This is a 13-mile loop. These marked bike routes are explained on a kiosk at the campground.

Hikers and bikers can enjoy the Two Lick Run Trail that starts at the front of the campground. It is a 4.6-mile pathway that climbs up Middle Mountain and swings around the head of the Two Lick watershed to make a loop. A shorter 1.8-mile loop uses the Two Lick Bottom Trail and part of the Two Lick Run Trail.

The nearby Laurel Creek Trail leaves Rimel Picnic Area, back on WV 39. The trail follows an old railroad grade to climb up and reach a backpacker's shelter at 5 miles, then circles around the slopes of Lockridge Mountain, returning to the picnic area at mile 8.

Supplies can be had back in Marlinton. It is but 4 miles to the mineral springs at Minnehaha. Pocahontas is one place where you shouldn't let an occasional passing car ruin your tent-camping experience.

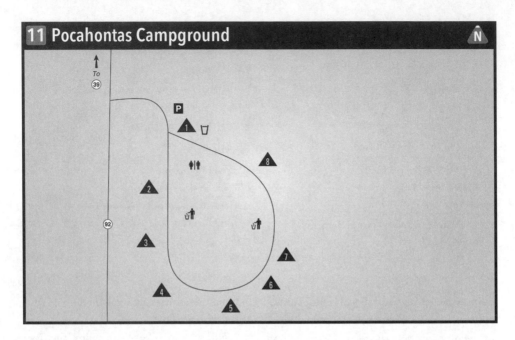

:: Getting There

From Marlinton, drive east on WV 39/92 for 13 miles to where WV 92 splits off to the right. Turn right on WV 92 south and follow it for 2 miles to Pocahontas Recreation Area, which will be on your left.

GPS COORDINATES N38° 06.153′   W79° 58.040′

12

Seneca State Forest

You will love the campground at West Virginia's oldest state forest.

Seneca is West Virginia's oldest state forest. It is also one of its quietest. Now, you can traverse the very hills and hollows that the Seneca Indians walked and enjoy some more-recent history at Cass Scenic Railroad State Park. Reenter the modern era with a visit to the National Radio Observatory in nearby Green Bank. Finally, return to the small campground set in a handsome hollow. No doubt, it is an odd collection of attractions in the area, but it allows you to appreciate the evolution of West Virginia through the generations.

You will also appreciate this campground. A Seneca ranger claims it is the finest in the state. He has a good case. The campground is set along a pair of small mountain streams. Rhododendron crowds the creeks. Overhead, a mixed forest of white pine, maple, and some oak shades the campsites. Steep hills stretch high around you.

The campsites are sheltered among the rhododendron away from the road. Camping areas have been leveled and set far apart from one another. Little bridges lead over the streams to most campsites, adding a certain quaintness to the natural beauty. Some campsites are heavily shaded by evergreens. Pass a vault toilet as you head toward the main hollow. Then the road forks up two small hollows. To the left is a road leading to two campsites. A grassy area lies between where the road splits. Here is the hand-pump well and two more vault toilets. Heavy rhododendron lies by the campsites along the creek. The road ends at a very private campsite. The Great Laurel Trail starts here.

The other road heads up the right-hand hollow. There are two more very private and secluded campsites that are the best in tent camping. This neat-as-a-pin, well-groomed campground has 10 sites; it could hold 20. However, even with its small numbers, it rarely, if ever, fills, making for a relaxing experience from the time you strike up your tent until you store it away in the trunk. Also of note is the coin-operated shower. This amenity is available behind the park office.

Trails for hikers and bikers lace the state forest. The Horseshoe Trail leaves the campground and makes a 1.5-mile loop. The Great Rhododendron Trail, named after the West Virginia state flower, leads a half mile from the campground to connect to the Hilltop Trail, one of many other paths around. The long-running Allegheny Trail meanders through the forest and has a trail shelter for overnight campers. The Fire Tower Trail leads to great views.

:: Ratings

BEAUTY: ★ ★ ★ ★ ★
PRIVACY: ★ ★ ★ ★
SPACIOUSNESS: ★ ★ ★ ★ ★
QUIET: ★ ★ ★ ★
SECURITY: ★ ★ ★ ★
CLEANLINESS: ★ ★ ★ ★ ★

:: Key Information

ADDRESS: Seneca State Forest, Route 1, Box 140, Dunmore, WV 24934

OPERATED BY: West Virginia State Parks

CONTACT: 304-799-6213, senecastateforest.com

OPEN: April–early December

SITES: 10

SITE AMENITIES: Picnic table, fire grate, tent pad

ASSIGNMENT: First come, first served; no reservations

REGISTRATION: Self-registration on-site

FACILITIES: Coin-operated shower, vault toilet, hand-pump well

PARKING: At campsites only

FEE: $12 per night

ELEVATION: 2,600 feet

RESTRICTIONS:

- **Pets:** On leash only
- **Fires:** In fire grates only
- **Alcohol:** Prohibited
- **Vehicles:** Two per site
- **Other:** 14-day stay limit

Many trails and back roads are open to mountain bikers. The Loop Road leads up toward the fire tower and past the shelter along the Allegheny Trail. Just 5 miles away is the Greenbrier River Trail, a long-distance rail trail that parallels the Greenbrier River, where there are also angling opportunities. On park property you can fish 4-acre Seneca Lake. It has trout, bass, and bluegill in its clear waters.

A West Virginia State Park highlight is the Cass Scenic Railroad, built in 1902. The train, an authentic locomotive with logging flatcars made into passenger coaches, leaves the restored town of Cass and climbs up the mountains to open fields and later to Whitaker Station. Then you can head up to Bald Knob, the second-highest point in the state at 4,842 feet. Enjoy great views from the overlook here. To reach Cass, leave north on WV 28 at the campground and follow the signs.

Also of interest is the National Radio Astronomy Observatory. It has been the focal point of radio astronomy for decades. Daily guided tours are offered Memorial Day–Labor Day. You can see science at work and observe how we learn about the world beyond our world. Self-guided walking and bicycling tours of the observatory can be taken any time of year. Head north on WV 28 from the campground and follow the signs to the observatory near Cass. After touring the observatory, you can enjoy your down-to-earth campground at Seneca State Forest.

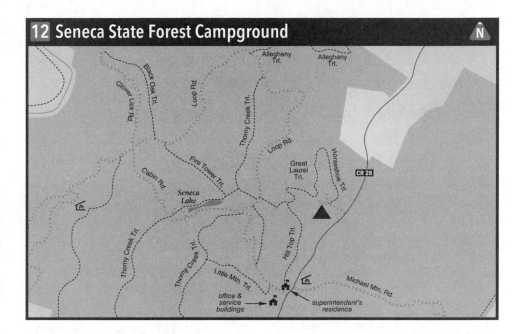

:: Getting There

From Marlinton, drive east on WV 39 for 5 miles to WV 28. Turn left on WV 28 and follow it 11 miles north to Seneca State Forest.

GPS COORDINATES N38° 18.397' W79° 55.331'

13

Spruce Knob Lake

The highest campground in this book lies near the highest point in the state.

Spruce Knob is a component of the Spruce Knob–Seneca Rocks National Recreation Area. This is the land of superlatives: the highest campground in the state, the highest lake in the state, and the highest point in the state. The surrounding mountains are laced with trails that traverse the forests, fields, and streams. Campers can enjoy the cool air of the high country at drive-up campsites or walk-in tent campsites.

Regardless of your point of entry, it is a good drive through rugged terrain to reach the campground. Bring all supplies you will need. Enter the paved campground loop and drive uphill through a northern hardwood forest. This deciduous woodland, perched at 4,000 feet, will be one of the last places to leaf out and one of the first places to turn colorful in the state.

Begin to pass campsites tucked away in deep woods off the loop road. The understory is thick here, which is good for campsite privacy. The sites are average in size and have numerous combinations of sun and shade, though most are on the shady side.

:: Ratings

BEAUTY: ★ ★ ★ ★
PRIVACY: ★ ★ ★ ★
SPACIOUSNESS: ★ ★ ★
QUIET: ★ ★ ★ ★ ★
SECURITY: ★ ★ ★
CLEANLINESS: ★ ★ ★ ★

The hill you climb is pretty steep, but the campsites have been leveled. This vertical variation adds beauty and privacy to already secluded campsites. The hill tops out at campsite 20. Additional attractive campsites are spread out along both sides of the road as it heads back down the mountainside.

Make a sharp left turn and the campground road runs perpendicular to the slope of the mountain. Along here are many walk-in sites that will appeal to tent campers. Wooden steps lead up or down to the spots that are just a short walk into the woods. Campers park parallel to the loop road.

Vault toilets and pump wells are spread throughout the campground. There is a solar-powered well near campsite 20 that delivers water through a spigot. Spruce Knob Lake will fill on summer holidays. But it is not busy during spring, which can be cool, or after August, when the campground will be draped in fall's decorations. Freezing temperatures are a real possibility during the shoulder seasons.

You must check out the area's superlatives. First, make the short drive to the actual Spruce Knob. This is West Virginia's highest point, at 4,861 feet. The Whispering Spruce Trail encircles the observation tower, going through highland woods to open up on a rocky field with great views. Farther-reaching 360-degree views can be had from the tower.

:: Key Information

ADDRESS: Spruce Knob Lake Campground, HC 59, Box 240, Petersburg, WV 26847

OPERATED BY: U.S. Forest Service

CONTACT: 304-257-4488, **www.fs.usda .gov/mnf;** reservations 877-444-6777, **reserveamerica.com**

OPEN: Mid-April–early October

SITES: 30 drive-up sites, 12 walk-in tent sites

SITE AMENITIES: Picnic table, fire grate, lantern post, tent pad

ASSIGNMENT: First come, first served unless reserved

REGISTRATION: Self-registration on-site

FACILITIES: Vault toilets, pump well, solar water spigot

PARKING: At campsites and walk-in parking area

FEE: $12 per night walk-in tent sites, $14 drive-up sites

ELEVATION: 4,000 feet

RESTRICTIONS:

■ **Pets:** On leash only

■ **Fires:** In fire grates only

■ **Alcohol:** At campsites only

■ **Vehicles:** None

■ **Boats:** No gas motors

■ **Other:** 14-day stay limit

Spruce Knob Lake is an attractive impoundment and offers good views from the water looking toward Spruce Knob. No gas motors are allowed on the 25-acre lake. Take your self-propelled boat to angle for rainbow trout and some bass. If fishing from the bank, use the 1-mile trail that encircles the lake. This walk is a pleasure for anyone, whether you fish or not. The Gatewood Trail makes a 2-mile loop and is connected to the campground by the Short Trail.

Hikers will also be interested in the Seneca Creek Backcountry. This primitive area lies just north of Forest Service Road 1 near the campground. There are streams, meadows, and views in the area. The most popular hike is the 5-mile trek to Upper Seneca Falls on the Seneca Creek Trail. The Allegheny Mountain Trail follows the backbone ridge of the area. The Lumberjack Trail leads out to the High Meadows Trail, where there are great views. All in all, 70 miles of paths traverse this country. The national forest produces a downloadable trail map of the Seneca Creek Backcountry. That should keep you more than busy during your stay at Spruce Knob Lake.

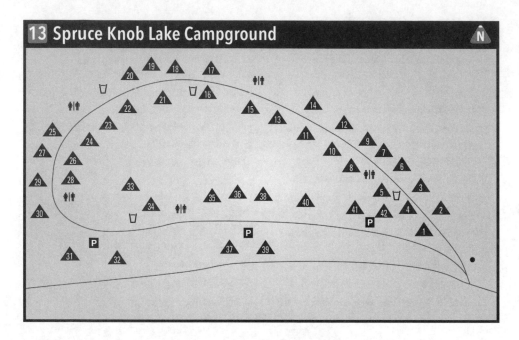

:: Getting There

From Seneca Rocks, drive south 10 miles to the hamlet of Cherry Grove and WV 28. Turn right on WV 28 and follow it 3 miles to Sawmill Run Road (CR 28/10). Turn right on Sawmill Run Road and follow it 8.4 miles to FR 112. Turn right on FR 112 and follow it 0.6 mile to FR 1. Turn left on FR 1 and follow it 0.6 mile to Spruce Knob Lake Campground, which will be on your right.

GPS COORDINATES   N38° 42.460'   W79° 35.100'

14

Summit Lake

Summit Lake offers fine water recreation in the southwest Monongahela National Forest.

Summit Lake is an example of a well-developed recreation area, not as in overly developed, but developed to the point of making the area more user-friendly. The two forks of Coats Run once quietly dropped down to the North Fork Cherry River. Now they feed the impoundment of Summit Lake, which rests in a flat high above the North Fork Cherry River. A scenic hiking trail lies around Summit Lake, which is stocked for fishing. Other pathways comb the area and lead to the primitive Cranberry Backcountry, where there are more opportunities for hiking, fishing, and nature study. Beyond this lie still more Monongahela National Forest pursuits.

The name Summit Lake seems appropriate after the drive up from Richwood. Turn onto the paved campground road, pass the fee station, and enter the first of two loops. This loop has nine campsites, tiered and leveled into a mountainside.

Seven of the nine are on the inside of the loop. Each campsite pull-in is paved. Each graveled area houses a picnic table,

fire grate, and lantern post. The pebbles are a little tough to drive a tent stake into. Overhead are deciduous trees, such as tulip, sugar maple, beech, and oak. A set of vault toilets and a water spigot lie on the outside of the loop. A trail heads to Summit Lake from near the toilets.

The second loop, also paved, is farther up the main road. Twenty-four well-spaced campsites make this a much bigger loop. The campsites, mostly on the outside of the loop, with nice views into the surrounding woods, are also cut into the mountainside and leveled. Some of the campsites are pull-through. Others have picnic tables and camping areas just inside the woods for added privacy.

There are two pump wells on this loop, but the water I got tasted rusty. Get your water from the spigot at the first loop. There are two sets of vault toilets for each gender. A foot trail near the first set of bathrooms leads to Summit Lake.

Summit Lake is the center of the action around here—it is 42 acres of mountain-rimmed clarity. Beneath the surface swim all manner of fish: brook trout, brown trout, rainbow trout, largemouth bass, and crappie. Anglers can fish from the shore or get out on a boat. Electric motors and arm power are the only means of advancing your craft over the lake. Most bank-fishermen like to toss their lines in from the dam. There is also an all-access dock near the boat launch.

:: Ratings

BEAUTY: ★ ★ ★
PRIVACY: ★ ★ ★ ★
SPACIOUSNESS: ★ ★ ★
QUIET: ★ ★ ★ ★
SECURITY: ★ ★ ★
CLEANLINESS: ★ ★ ★ ★

:: Key Information

ADDRESS: Summit Lake Campground, Box 110, Richwood, WV 26261

OPERATED BY: U.S. Forest Service

CONTACT: 304-846-2695; www.fs.usda.gov/mnf

OPEN: April–November 30

SITES: 33

SITE AMENITIES: Picnic table, fire grate, lantern post

ASSIGNMENT: First come, first served; no reservations

REGISTRATION: Self-registration on-site

FACILITIES: Water spigot, pump well, vault toilets

PARKING: At campsites and visitor parking area

FEE: $10 per night

ELEVATION: 3,400 feet

RESTRICTIONS:

■ **Pets:** On leash only

■ **Fires:** In fire grates only

■ **Alcohol:** At campsites only

■ **Vehicles:** None

■ **Boats:** Electric motors only

■ **Other:** 14-day stay limit

The scenic aspects of the lake are best appreciated from the Summit Lake Trail. Start your hike near the boat put-in by an aspen tree, head north, and step over the two lake feeder streams. Turn back south and complete your 1.8-mile loop by crossing over the dam.

The second-best hike in the area is the Fisherman's Trail. This starts near the campground at the end of Forest Service Road 77, which starts just across from the turn into the campground. Drive the mile or so to the gate on FR 77 and come to a trailhead. To your left heading straight down is the Fisherman's Trail (231). This immediately drops down along Pleasant Hollow, arriving at the Cranberry River and a trail shelter in 1.5 miles. Here, you can hike and fish in either direction in the Cranberry Backcountry. There are 26,000 acres and more than 60 miles of trails to enjoy in this primitive area.

Also at the end of FR 77 is the Pocahontas Trail (263). To your left up a hill, it is 1.6 miles to Hanging Rock. You can return by the gated FR 99. To your right, it is 5 miles to Mikes Knob. There, the Pocahontas Trail connects to the end of gated FR 77 to the top of the mountain, where a fire tower once stood. Mountain bikers should note that FR 99 and FR 77 make excellent rides, as do many other forest roads in the area. A map of the Monongahela National Forest really helps.

For folks in cars, the best ride is the Highland Scenic Highway, aka WV 39/55. You drove a portion of the road from Richwood. Continue the drive up to Cranberry Visitor Center (worth a stop), and turn left on WV 150, which is the continuation of the scenic highway. Along the way are many overlooks. Two trails of note here are the High Rocks Trail, which has a great view, and the Black Mountain Loop, which has views, solitude, and history.

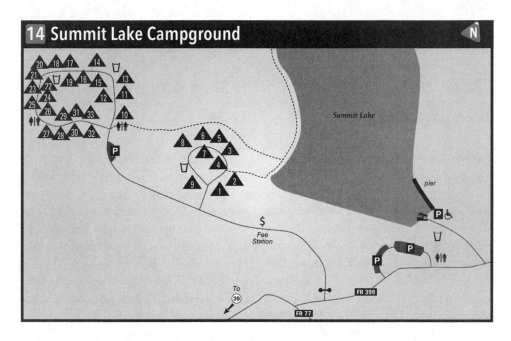

:: Getting There

From Richwood, drive east on WV 39/55 for 7.2 miles to Summit Lake Road (CR 39/5). Turn left on Summit Lake Road and climb for 2.1 miles to Summit Lake Campground.

GPS COORDINATES   N38° 14.866′   W80° 26.208′

15

Tea Creek

Tea Creek is at the center of many Monongahela National Forest attractions.

Tea Creek Campground used to be an old logging camp. A lot of hard labor went on here many decades ago. Now you can come here to escape the working world. And it is no job finding fun things to do. The nearby Williams River is a mecca for trout fishing, and hikers can trek the many trails of the Tea Creek Backcountry or the Cranberry Wilderness. The Highland Scenic Highway makes a great driving trip spring, summer, or fall. Tea Creek has had some flooding problems in the past. However, do not let this deter you. Just don't come if heavy rains are expected.

Cross the low-water bridge over Williams River and enter the Tea Creek Recreation Area. Just across the bridge are trailheads leading into the Tea Creek Backcountry. To your right is a spur road with several campsites strewn along Tea Creek. Most of the sites are not directly creekside, but five sites are along the rushing brook. The birch, maple, and tulip tree woods here are thick in spots, with an understory of rhododendron and small trees availing good campsite privacy. The sites here are large and spacious.

:: Ratings

BEAUTY: ★ ★ ★
PRIVACY: ★ ★ ★ ★
SPACIOUSNESS: ★ ★ ★ ★
QUIET: ★ ★ ★ ★
SECURITY: ★ ★ ★ ★
CLEANLINESS: ★ ★ ★ ★

Pass the campground host, and come to the road to your left. It is a loop circling through more dense woods. The woods are so thick that campsites are not visible to one another, whether they are on the inside or outside of the loop. I recommend this loop over the other road.

Expect to have company here on summer weekends. Get here early on Saturday mornings to make sure you get a campsite. During the week campsites are available in spring, summer, or fall. It gets a lot of local use on summer holidays.

Why do locals like Tea Creek? For starters, the Williams River flows right by the campground. Flowing for 22 miles through the national forest, it is a good fishery with catch-and-release sections, as well as catch-and-keep sections, where you can vie for rainbow, brown, and brook trout. Anglers will fish right from the bridge over the campground.

The Tea Creek Backcountry has an extensive network of trails that extend north from the campground. There are 40 miles of pathways. If you want to hike and fish, take the Williams Creek Trail, which heads upstream for 3 miles. Or you can walk upstream along Tea Creek, named for its reddish waters, for 3 miles, then turn right on the North Face Trail, climbing into the high country to reach the Tea Creek Mountain Trail at 6 miles. It is 1.5 more miles back down to reach the Williams Creek Trail near the campground, coming in at a little more

:: Key Information

ADDRESS: Tea Creek Campground, P.O. Box 210, Marlinton, WV 24954

OPERATED BY: U.S. Forest Service

CONTACT: 304-799-4334, **www.fs.usda.gov/mnf**

OPEN: April–November

SITES: 28

SITE AMENITIES: Picnic table, fire rings, lantern post

ASSIGNMENT: First come, first served; no reservations

REGISTRATION: Self-registration on-site

FACILITIES: Hand-pump water, vault toilet

PARKING: At campsites only

FEE: $10 per night

ELEVATION: 2,950 feet

RESTRICTIONS:

■ **Pets:** On leash only

■ **Fires:** In fire rings only

■ **Alcohol:** At campsites only

■ **Vehicles:** None

than 7 miles. Take this loop and you'll be ready for a dip in the cool waters of the Williams River.

You can also make a loop with the Bannock Shoals Run Trail, the Saddle Loop Trail, and the Turkey Point Connector Trail. This loop also covers the highs and lows of the mountainous surroundings and is around 9 miles. The Bannock Shoals Run Trail starts in the rear of the campground spur road.

You may feel like enjoying the mountains from your automobile. This is the place to do it. The Highland Scenic Highway runs right by Tea Creek. There are several overlooks and picnic areas along the 45-mile road. Head south and you can get great views to the east of the lands below the Allegheny Plateau. To your right is the Cranberry Wilderness. Several trails spur off the scenic highway into the Cranberry. One trail of note (High Rocks Trail) actually goes west, instead of east, into the Cranberry Wilderness. It is a 3-mile round-trip to a fantastic lookout on a rock outcrop. This well-marked trailhead is 10 miles south of Forest Service Road 86 at Tea Creek on the scenic highway.

Also worth a visit is the Cranberry Mountain Visitor Center, which offers more information and has descriptive nature displays. It is 13 miles south of the Tea Creek Area on the scenic highway. With a road this tempting to drive, you may be making a few supply runs into Marlinton just to get more views.

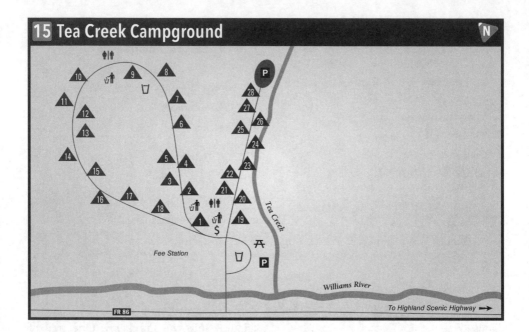

:: Getting There

From Marlinton, drive north on US 219 for 7 miles to Highland Scenic Highway. Turn left on Highland Scenic Highway and follow it south 10 miles to FR 86. Turn left on FR 86 and follow it a short distance to Tea Creek Campground, which will be on your right.

GPS COORDINATES   N38° 20.473'   W80° 13.933'

16

Watoga State Park

Watoga was one of West Virginia's first state parks.
It is still one of the finest.

There is so much going on at (and around) Watoga State Park, the state's largest, it is hard to describe it all. First, there is the natural scenery: Appalachian Mountains in their glory, carved by tumbling streams and the Greenbrier River, and a clear valley stream along which runs the famed Greenbrier River Trail. Add to that all the birds, mammals, and fish that call such settings home. The adjacent Calvin Price State Forest essentially doubles the size of the area.

Then there are the recreation opportunities: hiking, horseback riding, swimming, tubing, mountain biking, fishing, nature programs, and organized sports on several game courts. There are educational opportunities too. You can check out a little park history at the Civilian Conservation Corps Museum. Or learn about trees at the Brooks Arboretum. Three camping areas complete the Watoga picture. There are two separate campgrounds and one more-primitive camping area. Each offers a setting where any camper would be proud to pitch a tent.

:: Ratings

BEAUTY: ★ ★ ★
PRIVACY: ★ ★ ★
SPACIOUSNESS: ★ ★ ★
QUIET: ★ ★ ★ ★
SECURITY: ★ ★ ★ ★ ★
CLEANLINESS: ★ ★ ★ ★ ★

Beaver Creek is the original campground. Pass the check-in station and come to a camping area on your left. Several electric sites are set beneath a grassy woodland in a flat. They are of adequate size but a little close together. Farther back are larger, more secluded sites. A small playground and bathhouse are in the loops back here.

Straight ahead on the main road are five nice sites in a more wooded area. Pass a gate and turn left. The 10 campsites on this road are the park ranger's favorites. Across from this road is an open field.

The Riverside Campground is adjacent to the Greenbrier River, far from Beaver Creek. There are 20 waterfront sites (among a total of 50 here) shaded with evergreens, white pine, and maple and bordered with rhododendron. There is more than ample shade, even though a few sites are very open. Two bathhouses offer plenty of showering places for campers.

Watoga has a complex reservation system that is hard to explain, much less understand. Call the park if you are interested in reserving a site here. Watoga will fill on summer holidays, but only Riverside Campground fills most summer weekends. It is easier to get a site at Beaver Creek, and Beaver Creek is nearer most park facilities, except for accessing the Greenbrier River and Greenbrier River Trail.

The Greenbrier River Trail is a 75-mile rail trail. Mountain bikers love it, as it

:: Key Information

ADDRESS: Watoga State Park, HC 82, Box 252, Marlinton, WV 24954

OPERATED BY: West Virginia State Parks

CONTACT: 304-799-4087, **watoga.com;** reservations 800-225-5982

OPEN: April–early December

SITES: 50 electric, 38 nonelectric

SITE AMENITIES: Most have picnic table, fire grate, lantern post, tent pad

ASSIGNMENT: Reservations accepted but not required

REGISTRATION: By phone or at campground check-in station

FACILITIES: Hot showers, water spigots, coin laundry

PARKING: At campsites only

FEE: $23 per night electric, $20 nonelectric

ELEVATION: 2,100 feet

RESTRICTIONS:

■ **Pets:** On leash only

■ **Fires:** In fire grates only

■ **Alcohol:** Prohibited

■ **Vehicles:** None

■ **Other:** 14-day stay limit

crosses numerous bridges and a couple of tunnels, while paralleling the Greenbrier River. Hikers and other nature enthusiasts use the trail too. Anglers cast for bass on the river. Tubes can be rented near the park at Jack Horner's Corner in Seebert for those hot summer days.

There are 40 miles of trails inside Watoga, including a portion of the Allegheny Trail, which runs the length of the state. Enjoy great views of the Greenbrier River on the Arrowhead Trail atop the Ann Bailey Lookout Tower. Your most informative trails will be in the Brooks Arboretum area. These trails feature interpretive displays that enhance your knowledge of the woods. Of course, you can get information firsthand at Watoga during some of the programs that are held daily Memorial Day–Labor Day. Also, there are guided horse rides every day throughout the summer months.

Killbuck Lake offers 11 acres of boating and fishing. Rowboats and paddleboats are for rent; bass, bluegill, and trout occupy the lake for anglers. Many folks enjoy the water at the park pool. There is a recreation hall for rainy days. You can play tennis, table tennis, croquet, badminton, horseshoes, shuffleboard, and more, using park equipment. Come to think of it, with all that is offered, you may have to stay here a long time to do everything.

:: Getting There

From Marlinton, drive south 10 miles on US 219 to Seebert Road (CR 27). Turn left on Seebert Road and follow it 2 miles to Watoga State Park.

GPS COORDINATES   N38° 06.089'   W80° 05.605'

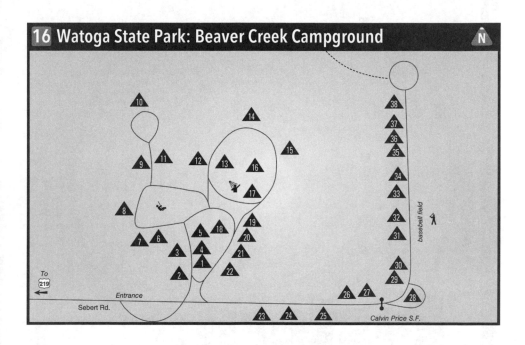

16 Watoga State Park: Beaver Creek Campground

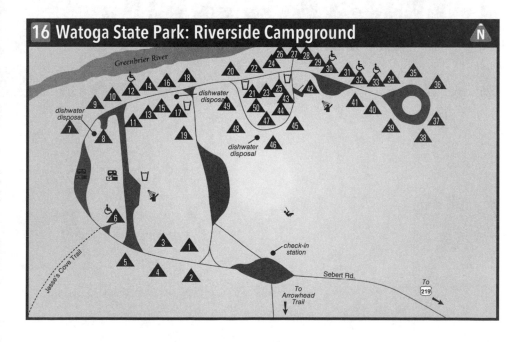

16 Watoga State Park: Riverside Campground

Eastern Panhandle

17

Big Bend

Camp down in the canyon of the Smoke Hole.

This campground lies in a dramatic setting. It is perched on a peninsula, with the South Branch Potomac River nearly encircling the camping area. On the outside of the river, wooded cliffs rise to form a natural cathedral. Old-timers called this the Smoke Hole because the mist rising from the deep gorge reminded them of smoke emerging from a cavity in the ground. The South Branch Potomac River attracts anglers vying for trout and smallmouth bass. Around the campground you'll see folks fiddling with rods, hanging up waders, and telling fishing tales. But even if you don't like to fish, this is a great destination. The setting can hardly be beat, and trails leave the campground and nearby vicinity. The campground itself is attractive and heavy on campsite privacy.

The drive here is "gorge-ous" and Big Bend only gets better. Enter the campground and look above at the mountain wall around you. Turn left, pass the campground host, and come to the River Loop. An old cemetery is off to your right, encircled by a wood fence. The River Loop is set in a plain along the river. It was once a field and is growing up in white pine, sycamore, autumn olive, and

a hodgepodge of other forest trees. Campsites are very dispersed. The forest service is keeping the area naturalized; many small trees and bushes provide dense cover and campsite privacy. The riverside campsites don't offer direct views of the river. However, the gorge is visible all around you.

The Upper Loop climbs the main road onto a hill. There are actually two loops. Enter the first loop, which has 17 campsites. White pines and autumn olive grow in great abundance here too. Locust trees also indicate this was a former field. But what you'll notice is that the density of the forest allows views of your campsite only.

The sites up here do not have tent pads, but just like the sites below, there are water spigots everywhere and a nice bathhouse for your convenience. The forest is thick, but the grass around the campsites is mowed regularly. The strange mix of trees here ranges from balsam to cedar to redbud. Some of the sites are set far back from the road.

The second upper loop is the highest and farthest from the river. It is much like the first upper loop. The dense, mixed forest continues. Campsite 39 is the very apex of the campground; land drops off all around it. From this point, it is downhill for the remainder of the loop.

Fishing is a big draw here. The South Branch Potomac River is a good fishery, but even if you get skunked, the music of the river and the sight of the Smoke Hole are keepers. There are other ways to enjoy the river. Canoeing is a great way to get on

:: Ratings

BEAUTY: ★ ★ ★ ★ ★
PRIVACY: ★ ★ ★
SPACIOUSNESS: ★ ★ ★ ★
QUIET: ★ ★ ★ ★
SECURITY: ★ ★ ★ ★
CLEANLINESS: ★ ★ ★ ★

:: Key Information

ADDRESS: Big Bend Campground, HC 59, Box 240, Petersburg, WV 26847

OPERATED BY: U.S. Forest Service

CONTACT: 304-257-4488, **www.fs.usda .gov/mnf;** reservations 877-444-6777, **reserveamerica.com**

OPEN: Mid-May–mid-October

SITES: 46

SITE AMENITIES: Picnic table, fire grate, lantern post; River Loop also has tent pad

ASSIGNMENT: First come, first served unless reserved

REGISTRATION: Online, by phone, or with campground host

FACILITIES: Water, hot showers, flush toilets

PARKING: At campsites only

FEE: (River Loop) $21 per night; (Upper Loop) $20 per night

ELEVATION: 1,200 feet

RESTRICTIONS:

■ **Pets:** On leash only

■ **Fires:** In fire rings only

■ **Alcohol:** At campsites only

■ **Vehicles:** None

■ **Other:** 14-day stay limit

the water and be right in the middle of the Smoke Hole Canyon. Eagle's Nest Outfitters, just outside Petersburg and in business for more than 20 years, specializes in river trips on the South Branch Potomac River, ranging from one hour to several days. Some river runs are dependent upon water levels. Contact them at 304-257-2393 or **eaglesnest outfitters.com** for more information.

Closer to your campsite is the Big Bend Loop Trail. It makes a 1-mile circle around the river and over the hill behind the campground. Anglers and bird-watchers enjoy the canyon views. The chimney you pass is the remnant of an old post office. Another nearby hike is South Branch Trail, a 3.5-mile loop that starts at the Smoke Hole Picnic Area, which you passed on the way in. Follow the river downstream; cut back up the ridge, passing fields and an old homestead; and then drop back down to the picnic area. Good views of the Smoke Hole Canyon can be found here, and this is what the Big Bend experience is all about.

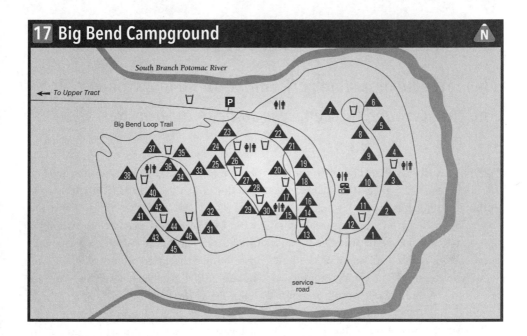

17 Big Bend Campground

South Branch Potomac River

← To Upper Tract

Big Bend Loop Trail

service road

:: Getting There

From Petersburg, drive south on US 220 for 12 miles to CR 2, which is just after a bridge crossing over South Branch Potomac River. Turn right on CR 2 and follow it 9 miles until it dead-ends at Big Bend Campground.

GPS COORDINATES   N38° 53.368'   W79° 14.331'

18

Blackwater Falls State Park

This is the highest state park campground in the book.
And the surrounding scenery is some of the best too.

This could be called high livin' in the high country. Take the panoramic Potomac Highlands, with its cold, clear rivers, open fields offering mountain vistas, and dense spruce-fir woodlands, and carve a state park out of some of the best scenery in the state. The campground itself is nothing to shout about from the mountaintops, but the mountaintop landscape will leave you breathless. It has the park's namesake waterfall, awesome views into the Blackwater River Canyon, good hiking and biking, and other amenities that are more down-to-earth.

Let's start with the campground. It is high and cool. Bring an extra sweater and a warm sleeping bag, even in the summer. Most nights will bring you closer to the campfire, especially in spring and fall.

The campground is divided into two loops. The right-hand loop has electricity. This means bigger rigs, but on my visit there weren't many. Twenty of these 30 sites can be reserved. This loop is set on a plateau forest of northern hardwoods in an area that is open and grassy. The first few sites are well wooded, but the latter half of the loop is very open, which can mean lots of sun and wind exposure. In the center of this loop is the heated bathhouse. Water spigots are set throughout the campground. The sites are not especially spacious or level, but there are a few desirable sites.

The left-hand loop has more vertical variation, yet it surprisingly has more good sites. The beginning of the loop slopes down but then rises back up. Most campsites have enough woods around them for adequate shade and privacy, but I wouldn't want to spend the night fighting gravity on some of these sloping sites. Be picky and you can get a good one. The last half of the loop is much more level, as is evidenced by the many disabled-accessible sites near the unheated bathhouse. All the sites on this loop, the loop most tent campers prefer, are first come, first served. Blackwater Falls fills on major summer holidays and an average of every other weekend during the summer, depending on the weather.

Your first stop should be the park's namesake. There are two ways to view it. Take the Gentle Trail a short distance, or take the trail from the Trading Post, a souvenir shop. Either way, the 65-foot falls will make you want more canyon scenery. You can see the Falls of Ekakala and a shot of the Blackwater River Canyon from Ekakala Trail. The Ekakala Trail starts near the park

:: Ratings

BEAUTY: ★ ★ ★
PRIVACY: ★ ★ ★
SPACIOUSNESS: ★ ★ ★
QUIET: ★ ★ ★ ★
SECURITY: ★ ★ ★ ★ ★
CLEANLINESS: ★ ★ ★ ★ ★

:: Key Information

ADDRESS: 1584 Blackwater Lodge Road, P.O. Drawer 490, Davis, WV 26260

OPERATED BY: West Virginia State Parks

CONTACT: 304-259-5216, blackwaterfalls.com

OPEN: Late April–October

SITES: 65

SITE AMENITIES: Picnic table, fire grate, lantern post. River Loop also has tent pad.

REGISTRATION: By phone or at campground registration station

ASSIGNMENT: First come, first served unless reserved

FACILITIES: Hot showers, flush toilets, coin laundry

PARKING: At campsites only

FEE: $23 per night electric, $20 nonelectric

ELEVATION: 3,100 feet

RESTRICTIONS:

■ **Pets:** On leash only

■ **Fires:** In fire rings only

■ **Alcohol:** At campsites only

■ **Vehicles:** None

■ **Other:** 14-day stay limit; one tent per site

lodge, where you can dine in style after your evening stroll. Make the short walk to Pendleton Point for a view of the lower canyon. The Balanced Rock Trail goes to an odd rock formation where one rock looks like it is a single rock balancing on top of another rock. Get a trail map from the campground registration station.

Many campers like to bike around the park and environs. Some backcountry trails allow bikes, but the park roads are really fun—and easier. If you want some challenging biking, try the Canaan Loop Road, which leaves the park and enters the Monongahela National Forest. The gravel road itself is fun to ride, and other trails spur off it. The road is open to vehicles, but I wouldn't bother unless I had a four-wheel-drive vehicle on

the section closest to Blackwater Falls. The Blackwater River offers both catch-and-keep and special catch-and-release fishing. The Department of Natural Resources stocks the canyon by helicopter. That is a sight to see.

Man-made diversions include swimming Pendleton Lake, where there is a beach that is open Memorial Day–Labor Day. You can fish it, too, for bass and bluegill. There are tennis, volleyball, and basketball courts in the vicinity. Also, near this area is the park's Nature Center. During summer months, the park offers daily nature and recreation programs led by a naturalist. Take advantage of this. You can learn a lot from a naturalist, knowledge that will enhance your appreciation for the Potomac Highlands and Blackwater Falls State Park.

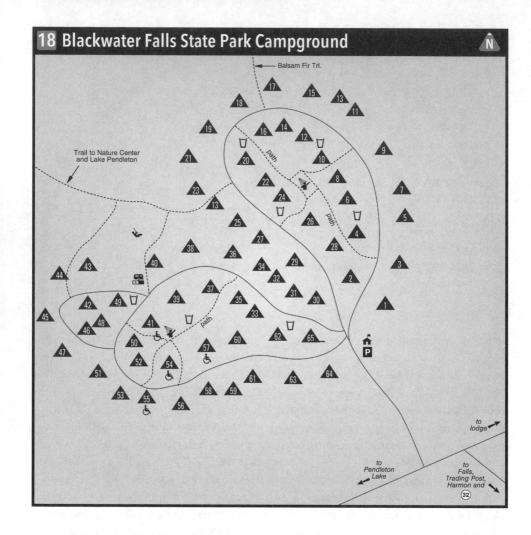

:: Getting There

From Harmon, drive north on WV 32 for 20 miles to the town of Davis. Once in Davis, turn left at the sign for Blackwater Falls and soon enter the park.

GPS COORDINATES   N39° 06.872'   W79° 29.310'

19

Brandywine Lake

Brandywine Lake is a fully developed national forest facility that has received a makeover. Now it's even better.

The town of Brandywine, 3 miles from the campground, benefits from this campground and recreation area. A great location for camping, hiking, and fishing, the town might not even be here if it weren't for the tall dam that forms Brandywine Lake. Water has reached the brim of the dam twice since 1964, when it was built. That might not seem impressive until you see how high the dam is in comparison to the size of Brandywine Lake. But don't let potential flooding scare you away. Any slice of flat ground in West Virginia—and there aren't many in the Mountain State—is capable of flooding.

Enter the attractive Hawes Run valley. The big dam and pretty lake will be on your right. The white sand beach contrasts well with the green grass of the picnic area. Pass by the new bathhouse and enter the camping area proper, set alongside Hawes Run. The lines of development are crisp and clean with the makeover, and they mesh well with the woodland. The paved loop road and paved pull-ins make the campground less dusty. Landscaping timbers delineate the

large, level graveled sites, which act as an oversize tent pad for your entire camping area. Overhead, a white pine–dominated forest lends plenty of shade. Numerous immature trees act as campsite barriers. The main road divides, then comes together, and seven ultralarge campsites are spread far apart here.

There is one more bathhouse and two more vault toilets. Plenty of water spigots are dispersed about. More campsites are laid out along Hawes Run. The hollow widens with the addition of a side branch. The camping area also widens and makes a final loop. These are the best sites. At the head of this loop is a grassy field that houses the group camp and overflow campsites.

No reservations are accepted here, which is unusual for a national forest campground this nice. However, barring major holidays, you should get a campsite if you arrive on a Friday before 6 p.m. Getting a site is no problem during the week. After October 1, services are reduced to only pump well water and vault toilets (prices are reduced accordingly). A trailer dump station may attract a few big rigs, but don't let that bother you. The lack of electricity, sewage hookups, and reservations keeps their numbers way down.

The dam-to-lake size ratio will impress you, but so will Brandywine Lake itself. It is a 10-acre clear impoundment backed against Cowger Mountain. Attractive picnic areas are near the lake. On summer days, adults

:: Ratings

BEAUTY: ★ ★ ★ ★
PRIVACY: ★ ★ ★ ★
SPACIOUSNESS: ★ ★ ★ ★ ★
QUIET: ★ ★ ★ ★
SECURITY: ★ ★ ★ ★
CLEANLINESS: ★ ★ ★ ★

:: Key Information

ADDRESS: Brandywine Lake,
112 North River Road,
Bridgewater, VA 22812

OPERATED BY: U.S. Forest Service

CONTACT: 540-432-0187,
www.fs.usda.gov/gwj

OPEN: Mid-May–mid-November

SITES: 34

SITE AMENITIES: Picnic table, fire grate,
tent pad, lantern post

ASSIGNMENT: First come, first served;
no reservations

REGISTRATION: Self-registration on-site

FACILITIES: Hot showers, flush toilets,
vault toilets, water spigots

PARKING: At campsites only

FEE: $16 per night

ELEVATION: 2,000 feet

RESTRICTIONS:

■ **Pets:** On leash only

■ **Fires:** In fire grates only

■ **Alcohol:** At campsites only

■ **Vehicles:** None

■ **Boats:** No gas motors

■ **Other:** 14-day stay limit

lounge by the beach, watching the kids play. Others fish for trout around the lake. No gas motors are allowed on the water.

Brandywine has an excellent hiking loop trail that is the right distance for nearly all tent campers. The 3.6-mile Sawmill Trail leaves the upper camping loop and makes a loop of its own. Parallel Hawes Run, crossing it four times and passing the site of a sawmill at mile 1.1. Cross Hawes Run one more time before winding across a couple of low ridges and circling some clearings. These clearings are wildlife food plots. When clearings are made, this creates "edges," places where two plant habitats meet. These edges are richer in food sources for wildlife than either of the two habitats individually. Make this 3.6-mile loop in the morning, and you may see wildlife, such as turkeys or deer, near one of these edges.

Most people come to Brandywine for the mountain-rimmed lake and its offerings. There might not be many people around here, including nearby residents, if it weren't for the lake. The folks in Brandywine are glad it's here; you will be too.

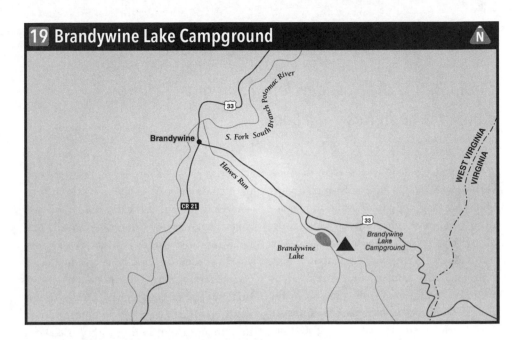

19 Brandywine Lake Campground

:: Getting There

From the town of Brandywine, turn east on US 33 and follow it 3 miles to Brandy-wine Recreation Area, which will be on your right.

GPS COORDINATES   N38° 35.935'   W79° 12.082'

20

Camp Run

Camp Run is the least developed and most primitive campground in this guidebook.

Do you remember the old television show *Seinfeld?* Its premise was "a show about nothing." Apparently they did something because the show was on a long time. That could be the premise for Camp Run Campground. Camping here is about doing nothing. The campground is extremely primitive and rough—the gravel on the campground road is minimal, the campsites aren't numbered, there's no registration, there's no bulletin board of things to do, and there's no fee.

On the surface it does seem there is nothing to do here. Oh, you could fish Camp Run and Little Camp Run. Or you could fish Camp Run Lake below the campground. But why bother? Just come here and do nothing but perfect the lost art of true outdoor camping "1950s-style," as the national forest website states. True outdoor camping—where you overnight in a tent and enjoy the natural world around you by day—is possible even when the weather doesn't exactly cooperate. When it's cold, you perfect your fire-building techniques or grill out. When it's rainy, you get a tarp set up just right and play cards or read a book, every once in while looking out at the downpour and getting a laugh out of being satisfactorily dry. Or when the weather is ideal, you get out your tree identification book and finally set about learning what these big tall plants are that make you feel so relaxed. Or maybe it is finally getting to spend some uninterrupted time in a peaceful setting with those about whom you care most.

Camp Run has been a good place to pitch a tent for a long time, judging by its name. The camping area is set just below the confluence of Camp Run and Little Camp Run. A high mountainside looms to your right, and Camp Run flows along to your left. A level, pretty hollow runs up to the mountainside, and this is where the campsites lie. The 10 campsites, each with picnic table, concrete fire grate with a grill attached, lantern post, and tent pad, are far back from the road. Two sites on the small turnaround at the head of the campground are especially attractive. The oak-hickory-pine forest is tall overhead.

Vault toilets for each gender are the only amenities. The pump well has been capped. This is a remote park, without a campground host or regular visits by a ranger, so it's up to the users to keep the place clean. Please apply the "pack it in, pack it out" philosophy here.

People live in the nearby area, but it is a very isolated campground. Make sure to

:: Ratings

BEAUTY: ★ ★ ★ ★
PRIVACY: ★ ★ ★ ★
SPACIOUSNESS: ★ ★ ★
QUIET: ★ ★ ★ ★
SECURITY: ★ ★ ★
CLEANLINESS: ★ ★

:: Key Information

ADDRESS: Camp Run Campground, 112 North River Road, Bridgewater, VA 22812

OPERATED BY: U.S. Forest Service

CONTACT: 540-432-0187, www.fs.usda.gov/gwj

OPEN: Year-round

SITES: 10

SITE AMENITIES: Picnic table, fire grate, tent pad, lantern post

ASSIGNMENT: First come, first served; no reservations

REGISTRATION: None

FACILITIES: Vault toilets; bring water

PARKING: At campsites only

FEE: None

ELEVATION: 1,800 feet

RESTRICTIONS:
- **Pets:** On leash only
- **Fires:** In fire grates only
- **Alcohol:** At campsites only
- **Vehicles:** None
- **Other:** 14-day stay limit

bring in your supplies or you'll be running the roads back to Franklin. By the way, the valleys and mountains of this part of West Virginia are among the state's prettiest.

Fishing is the only thing you can do directly from the campground. But if you want to go hiking, head to Lost River State Park: Take Route 3 north to County Road 12. Turn right on CR 12 and follow this pretty road with lots of views over South Branch Mountain to the state park. They have more than 18 miles of trails there. You can also see the old Lee Cabin and eat at the park restaurant. They don't have a park-run campground. So you could hike at Lost River State Park. Or not. When I stayed at Camp Run, I did nothing, not a thing.

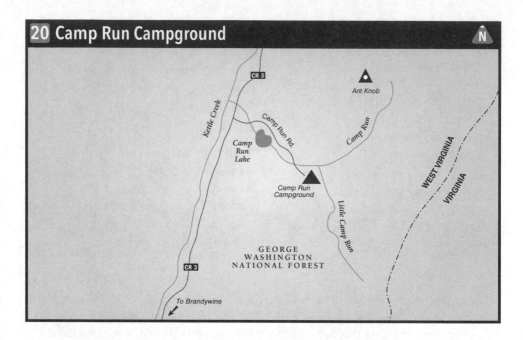

:: Getting There

From Brandywine, head north on US 33. Follow it 3.3 miles to Route 3 in Oak Flat. Turn right on Route 3 and follow it 10 miles to Route 3/1 (Camp Run Road). Follow the gravel road 1.5 miles, passing Camp Run Lake to Camp Run Campground, which will be on your right.

GPS COORDINATES   N38° 44.854′   W79° 06.559′

21

Hawk

It's hard to believe this campground is free.

Hawk lies in a remote corner of West Virginia in a remote corner of the George Washington National Forest. However, I found my way here. And when I pulled up to Hawk, my first thought was, "I can't believe this campground is free!" Then I made a loop, found a site, and began to enjoy an ideal spring day. Dogwoods, a major understory tree in this campground, were blooming everywhere. A profusion of creamy blossoms dotted the woodland. Overhead, the oak, maple, and hickory trees were just budding. This place is loaded with oaks— northern white, scarlet, and black. I got out my tree book and began to identify just how many oaks there were. The answer? A lot.

This is one of the nicest free national forest campgrounds I've seen anywhere. Situated in the northwesternmost slice of the George Washington National Forest, it seems to have been forgotten. But it hasn't been left to fall into disrepair. Quite the contrary: The campsites were just as good as a pay campground; the pump well and vault toilets were fine; the picnic area and group campground were also in good condition.

:: Ratings

BEAUTY: ★ ★ ★ ★
PRIVACY: ★ ★ ★ ★
SPACIOUSNESS: ★ ★ ★ ★ ★
QUIET: ★ ★ ★ ★ ★
SECURITY: ★ ★ ★
CLEANLINESS: ★ ★ ★ ★

Great North Mountain, the dividing line between West Virginia and Virginia, rises just a few miles east. Hawk is set on a flat of the mountain slope. A little stream runs nearby, but this is an upland forest with a western exposure, hence all the oaks. Enter the campground loop and pass the first of two vault toilets for each gender. Notice how the campsites are so large and well dispersed. Large stones delineate the parking areas. The tent pads are graveled for good drainage.

The first few sites have the least tree cover. Yet there is still adequate shade, except at high noon. The slope increases past campsite 6. However, a little stonework levels the parking and camping areas. The sites toward the end of the loop look down into the woods and are heavily shaded. A few sites are on the inside of the loop, but there really is not a bad site here.

Campsite use is little to nil during the week. Sites are available nearly every weekend, especially during cooler times of the year. Since the forest service garners no revenue from this campground, there is no garbage service. It is a "pack it in, pack it out" campground. Do your part to keep it as nice as when I spent my early May day here.

I suggest coming during the spring or fall. Summertime might be too hot at this 1,400-foot elevation, especially with no water to speak of nearby. Besides, the shoulder seasons are a good time to hike. And the Tuscarora Trail passes right by the campground. This is a long-distance trail that

:: Key Information

ADDRESS: Hawk Recreation Area, 109 Molineau Road, Edinburgh, VA 22834

OPERATED BY: U.S. Forest Service

CONTACT: 540-984-4101, www.fs.usda.gov/gwj

OPEN: Late April–December

SITES: 15

SITE AMENITIES: Picnic table, fire ring, lantern post, tent pad

ASSIGNMENT: First come, first served; no reservations

REGISTRATION: Self-registration on-site

FACILITIES: Pump well, vault toilets

PARKING: At campsites only

FEE: None

ELEVATION: 1,400 feet

RESTRICTIONS:

■ **Pets:** On leash only

■ **Fires:** In fire ring only

■ **Alcohol:** At campsites only

■ **Vehicles:** None

■ **Other:** 21-day stay limit

goes from Virginia to Pennsylvania via West Virginia. It was designed as an alternative long-distance trail to the Appalachian Trail.

Walk back to the campground entrance. Across the road is a blue-blazed trail. To your right, running by the picnic area, is also a blue-blazed trail. This is the Tuscarora. A right turn will take you downhill and downstream for a 1.5-mile walk to Hawk Run. There are some small falls along the stream. You can keep from backtracking by cutting west and returning up one of the gated roads back toward Hawk.

The most popular hike on the Tuscarora goes left (uphill), winding back and forth up the slope of Great North Mountain, reaching the crest at 1.8 miles. Keep on, crossing a couple of roads, then coming to a rock outcrop and view at 3.8 miles. If you continue, there is a trail shelter at 4.3 miles. A side trail descends to a spring here if you need water. This hike may or may not stimulate you to try such a walk for the length of the state. There is also another closer, shorter walk. The Margaret Gollady Wild Flower Trail leaves the campground near campsite 6. It was so new when I walked it that I couldn't follow it. I hope it is better marked by now.

Even as out-of-the-way as the campground feels, the town of Wardensville and its stores are just a few miles distant. Yet Wardensville seems like a world away from the oaks and dogwoods at Hawk.

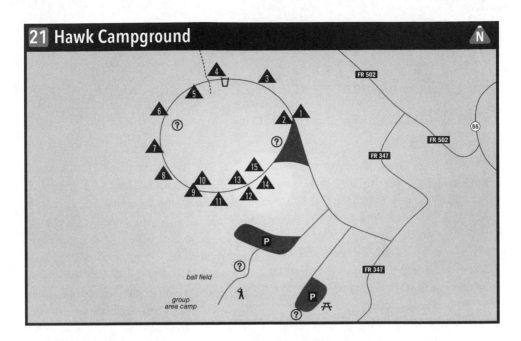

21 Hawk Campground

:: Getting There

From Wardensville, drive east on WV 55 for 4 miles. Turn left on FR 502 and follow it for 3 miles to FR 347, your first left. Continue 0.8 mile to Hawk Recreation Area, which will be on your right.

GPS COORDINATES N39° 06.969'   W78° 30.084'

22

Red Creek

*Red Creek is highland headquarters for exploring the Dolly
Sods Wilderness and Scenic Area.*

This is one of the highest campgrounds in the state—perched at nearly 4,000 feet, atop the same high plateau that houses the Dolly Sods. The flora and climate are more like Canada than West Virginia. On my trip here in early May, most of the trees had not yet begun to leaf out. It is a whole different world from the "lowlands" below. The air cools significantly as you drive up the plateau. Snow is a possibility here eight months of the year. Freezing temperatures can occur any time of year. This is not to scare you off; rather, Red Creek can be a refreshing break during the long, hot summer. But bring warm clothes all the same.

Maybe you can keep warm by hiking because the Dolly Sods is laced with trails. These trails pass through spruce thickets, northern hardwood forests, and many open areas known as plains. The forest here was once logged, and fires followed. In many areas the topsoil was burned to the rock below. These areas have remained treeless and add to the beauty and scenery. Vistas seem to be everywhere.

:: Ratings

BEAUTY: ★ ★ ★ ★
PRIVACY: ★ ★ ★
SPACIOUSNESS: ★ ★ ★
QUIET: ★ ★ ★ ★ ★
SECURITY: ★ ★ ★
CLEANLINESS: ★ ★ ★ ★

I like this campground. It is small and rustic. Campsites are well dispersed, and you can actually go hiking right from your tent. Two small creeks converge in the campground, which is in a northern hardwood forest. Cherry, yellow birch, red maple, serviceberry, beech, a few spruce, and aspens—a rarity this far south—adorn the area. The forest is fairly young, and many of the trees have a stunted look. Some campsites can be sunny at high noon.

Enter the loop, and the first campsite is wide open. But then you come to a parking area for two walk-in tent sites. Take a short path to these sites that are set apart from the rest of the campground. These are ideal for tent campers who want the most in privacy. Beyond this, the sites are well dispersed. Some are set far back from the road.

A small bridge connects campers in the back of the loop to the modern vault toilets in the center of the loop. The pump well is also here, toward the front of the loop. This small campground will fill on major holidays but is weather dependent; nice weekends can bring people out. Most campers here are active folks who want to explore the wealth of unusual West Virginia beauty around them.

The Dolly Sods Wilderness is 10,000 acres of exceptional country. The Dolly Sods Scenic Area is much the same as the adjoining wilderness. A great hike is the Blackbird Knob Trail, which starts just outside

:: Key Information

ADDRESS: Red Creek Campground, HC 59, Box 240, Petersburg, WV 26847

OPERATED BY: U.S. Forest Service

CONTACT: 304-257-4488, www.fs.usda.gov/mnf

OPEN: Mid-April–November

SITES: 12

SITE AMENITIES: Picnic table, fire ring, lantern post

ASSIGNMENT: First come, first served; no reservations

REGISTRATION: Self-registration on-site

FACILITIES: Pump well, vault toilets

PARKING: At campsites and walk-in tent camper parking area only

FEE: $11 per night

ELEVATION: 3,900 feet

RESTRICTIONS:

■ **Pets:** On leash only

■ **Fires:** In fire rings only

■ **Alcohol:** At campsites only

■ **Vehicles:** None

■ **Other:** 14-day stay limit

the campground. Take the path and head through some thick woods where great views soon open up to the mountains and plains around you. Cross Alder Branch and the Red Creek before emerging onto another flat field. Continue beyond this, passing the Red Creek Trail, which splits off to the left. Keep forward and skirt the edge of Blackbird Knob. Climb the open hill to your right amid a boulder field. There are stupendous views of the Red Creek gorge and the Allegheny Mountains stretching off to the southwest.

Just south of the campground is the Northland Loop Trail. It is a 0.4-mile interpretive trail that gives you an idea of the region's ecology. Back a ways on Forest Service Road 75 are several trails that enter Dolly Sods. The Rohrbaugh Plains Trail offers very good overlooks about 2 miles from the road. You can make a loop using the Rohrbaugh Plains Trail, the Wildlife Trail, and FR 75. The Red Creek Trail is the backbone of the trail system in the Dolly Sods. You can catch this trail from Blackbird Knob or drive south from the campground to Farm Route 19 toward Laneville and start your hike from the bottom up.

Actually, with this much open terrain, off-trail hiking is an option. But if you want to experience a different side of West Virginia, experience Dolly Sods and Red Creek Campground.

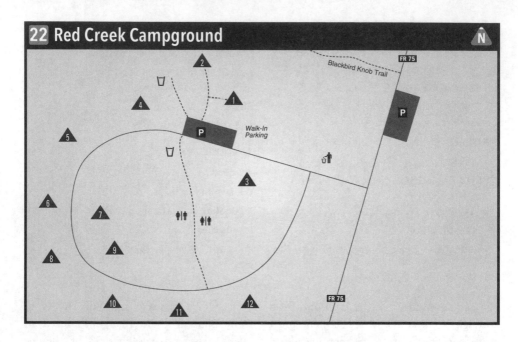

:: Getting There

From Petersburg, drive west on WV 28 for 8.5 miles to Jordan Run Road (CR 28/7). Turn right on Jordan Run Road and follow it 1 mile to FR 19, which will be on your left. Turn left on FR 19 and follow it 6 miles to FR 75. Turn right on FR 75 and follow it 5 miles to Red Creek, which will be on your left.

GPS COORDINATES   N39° 01.952′   W79° 18.888′

23

Seneca Shadows

The walk-in tent sites here have a majestic view of Seneca Rocks.

This is one of the forest service's better campgrounds, and they sure picked the right place to put it—the layout and facilities are perched on a hill with a million-dollar view of Seneca Rocks. This view is reserved for the walk-in tent sites only. The rest of the campground has to settle for a high-quality camping area adjacent to many forest activities and other nearby attractions. You are a winner no matter where you stay at Seneca Shadows.

Drive the paved road past the seldom-used registration station, and come to Loop A. Turn right and descend into an oak-hickory forest. Campsites are spread on either side of the road, which ends in a small turnaround. Even though the terrain is sloped, the campsites are not. The paved pull-ins are level, as are the gravel-and-sand tent pads. Some sites have wooden steps on them to access the tent pad or picnic table. Site spaciousness is no problem, and an understory of smaller trees and brush keeps the sites private. A fully equipped bathhouse with a water spigot completes the picture.

Loop B is much like Loop A, only it is farther down the main road. The campsites here are very dispersed, and the vertical variation between sites adds to the campsite privacy. Pass the road to the amphitheater and come to Loop C. This camping area splits off into two roads. The terrain is more level and the 13 campsites are equipped with electricity. There is a toilet and a bathhouse here.

Pass the group camp and come to the tent camper's parking area. Walk a short path to the far side of a row of trees and come to the tent campers' area in a level, grassy field. Off to your right, in plain view for every tent camper, are Seneca Rocks. Next to the row of trees is a row of tent sites. The center of the grassy field is left naturalized. Across this grass are more tent sites. Up on a hill to your left are a few sites that have the grandest view of them all. Down the hill are even more tent sites. Each of these 40 sites is well marked and delineated. A few trees dot the area. Planners just couldn't stand to wreck the view. And I understand.

There are vault toilets by the parking area. Showers are a short walk away in the bathhouse for Loop C. A covered pavilion in the tent camper's area is perfect for cooking on rainy days.

Looking at those rocks just drives folks to surmount them. There is a steep, 1.3-mile foot trail to Seneca Rocks, which rise 900 feet above the valley floor. The trail starts near the expanded visitor center, where there are interpretive displays and forest information.

:: Ratings

BEAUTY: ★ ★ ★ ★ ★
PRIVACY: ★ ★ ★
SPACIOUSNESS: ★ ★ ★ ★
QUIET: ★ ★ ★ ★
SECURITY: ★ ★ ★ ★ ★
CLEANLINESS: ★ ★ ★ ★ ★

:: Key Information

ADDRESS: Seneca Shadows, HC 59, Box 240, Petersburg, WV 26847

OPERATED BY: U.S. Forest Service

CONTACT: 304-257-4488, **www.fs.usda .gov/mnf;** reservations 877-444-6777, **reserveamerica.com**

OPEN: April 15–October 31

SITES: 13 electric, 65 nonelectric

SITE AMENITIES: Picnic table, fire ring, tent pad, lantern post

ASSIGNMENT: First come, first served unless reserved

REGISTRATION: By phone or with campground host

FACILITIES: Hot showers, flush and vault toilets, water spigots

PARKING: At campsites or tenter's parking area

FEE: $15 per night walk-in tent area, $20 nonelectric, $20 electric

ELEVATION: 1,600 feet

RESTRICTIONS:

■ **Pets:** On leash only

■ **Fires:** In fire rings only

■ **Alcohol:** At campsites only

■ **Vehicles:** None

■ **Other:** 14-day stay limit

There are also interpretive programs at the campground on summer weekends.

Rock climbers often stay at the campground so they can attack Seneca Rocks with ropes and harnesses and helmets. If you would like to rock climb, there is a rock climbing school a mile away in the town of Seneca Rocks. From April to October, learn to climb from Seneca Rocks Climbing School. Or if you have some experience, go on a guided climb. Their website is **seneca-rocks.com.**

If you don't want to climb, then head underground. Go on a guided tour of Seneca Caverns. See all the weird rock formations and Mirror Lake. This cavern is south of the campground on US 33. The whole area is pretty, and Seneca Rocks is especially scenic. If the views here don't inspire you, it's time to put the tent up for sale.

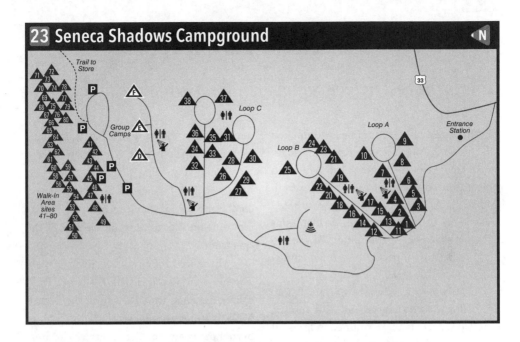

23 Seneca Shadows Campground

:: Getting There

From the town of Seneca Rocks, drive south on US 33 for 1.5 miles. The campground will be on your right.

GPS COORDINATES   N38° 49.417′   W79° 23.195′

24

Sleepy Creek WMA

This is the best in tent camping in West Virginia's far east.

This area of West Virginia is dominated by long north-south running ridges with valleys between them. You will learn this lesson well coming to Sleepy Creek from Martinsburg. Sleepy Creek Lake is situated in a narrow valley between Third Hill Mountain and Sleepy Creek Mountain. These two mountains are connected by a ridge named Lock-of-the-Mountain.

This was originally a state forest. Before that, it had been logged out and hunted out. Now, there is a lake rimmed in forested mountains filled with trails in the 23,000-acre area. The four campgrounds do not match the scenery, but they will do, especially for the price. Hiking and fishing are the main activities for most tent campers. Check with the wildlife manager for the best and safest times to enter the woods.

One of the major differences between a state forest and a wildlife management area is the primary reason they are managed. Most West Virginia state forests are managed for timber, then recreation. Most WMAs are managed for wildlife and hunting, then recreation. State parks are managed for preservation and recreation, not necessarily in that order. What this means for tent campers is that WMAs can be very scenic and rewarding places to camp and have fun. Just be careful about when you come, and know that the camping is liable to be on the more primitive end of the spectrum.

There are many trails at Sleepy Creek. The most prominent is the Tuscarora Trail, a long-distance trail that runs the length of the state. A 20-mile section of this blue-blazed pathway runs the length of the area. Sleepy Creek Lake, a long, narrow impoundment with many snags in it, is the area's centerpiece. Angling is a peaceful experience here, as no motors are allowed in the lake.

Drive down from Third Hill Mountain and come to the lake. The campground farthest to the right is the 22-site Lower Campground. This camp is set in a young forest on a knoll. The views here are pretty good, but the sun could dominate the camping experience, which could be good on a cool winter day.

The next campground is Piney Point near the lake. The first three campsites are in a field next to some woods. Next, overlooking the lake are several campsites that are too close together. There is one good solo site next to the lake.

The Myers Place Campground is near an old homesite. Drop off onto a spit of land jutting into the lake where some of the campsites are up on the hill and other campsites are beneath young woods by the lake.

:: Ratings

BEAUTY: ★ ★
PRIVACY: ★ ★ ★
SPACIOUSNESS: ★ ★ ★
QUIET: ★ ★ ★ ★ ★
SECURITY: ★ ★ ★
CLEANLINESS: ★ ★ ★

:: Key Information

ADDRESS: Sleepy Creek, 1910 Sleepy Creek Road, Hedgesville, WV 25427

OPERATED BY: West Virginia Division of Natural Resources

CONTACT: 304-754-3855, **www.wvdnr .gov/hunting/d2wmaareas.shtm**

OPEN: Year-round

SITES: 75

SITE AMENITIES: Fire ring, lantern post

ASSIGNMENT: First come, first served; no reservations

REGISTRATION: Self-registration on-site

FACILITIES: Vault toilets, hand-pump well

PARKING: At campsites only

FEE: $5 per night

ELEVATION: 1,100 feet

RESTRICTIONS:

■ **Pets:** On leash only

■ **Fires:** In fire rings only

■ **Alcohol:** Prohibited

■ **Vehicles:** 17-foot trailer limit

■ **Boats:** No motors

■ **Other:** 14-day stay limit

The 13-site Upper Campground has sunny and shady sites. The best campsites are several under the piney woods. The whole place has a primitive, rough look. With 75 total sites, it's possible get a campsite any day of the year. Bring in all your supplies, including water, though the Myers Spring is a potential source of liquid refreshment.

The Tuscarora Trail leaves on the gated road south from the Upper Campground. Here, you cross Roaring Run and can continue on the Roaring Run Trail to head uphill on the Tuscarora Trail. If you take the Tuscarora Trail the other way, pass the lake and campgrounds, and connect to other area trails that are just now being named and signed. Other trails designated for mountain bikers and equestrians are blazed in red.

The jewel of this place is the lake. There are 205 acres of water where mountains rise above and fish swim below. Bring your canoe, and paddle right from your campsite, if you get a lakeside spot. I was overwhelmed by the quiet early morning here. It was just the birds—no wind or anything. Anglers can vie for northern pike, largemouth bass, bluegill, and crappie. If you are bait fishing with a bobber, it will be hard to keep your eyes on the cork with the scenery around you.

24 Sleepy Creek WMA Campground

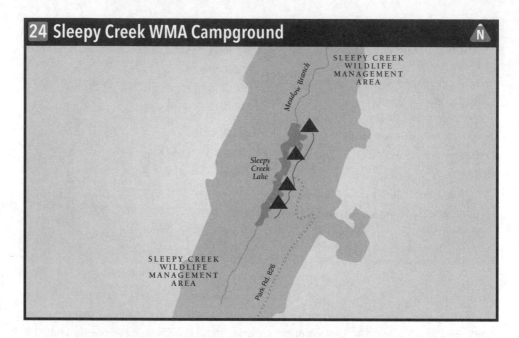

:: Getting There

From Exit 15 on I-81 in Martinsburg, take CR 13 west over North Mountain. The main paved road over the mountain changes to CR 15, then CR 18, but stay with the main road. Continue through the four-way stop at Shanghai, and climb Third Hill Mountain. After a total of 12 miles from Martinsburg, come to the sign for Sleepy Creek Lake at the top of the mountain. Turn right at Park Road (826) and follow it 5 miles to the lake.

GPS COORDINATES   N39° 30.827′   W78° 09.120′

25

Trout Pond

Trout Pond is West Virginia's only natural lake.
Some man-made amenities add to the setting.

West Virginia's only natural lake, Trout Pond is a water-filled sinkhole amid some of the state's prettiest country-side. This forest service recreation area was tastefully integrated into the setting. There are fun things to do here. The facilities are clean and well maintained, especially the campground. Once here, you will agree this corner of the Mountain State is worth at least one weekend of your life.

Trout Pond Campground is situated on a mountain flat in a pretty dry forest of oak, hickory, dogwood, and a few pine trees. Many small trees and brush give the impression that the campground was gently set into the woods, as opposed to the land being bulldozed, campsites laid out, and then a few trees planted. Some campgrounds are built that way. Not this one.

Drive into the loop. The first 10 sites are on both sides of the road and have electricity. Campsites are very well delineated and are bordered with landscaping timbers to keep the natural and camping areas separate. Pass the first of three modern bathhouses with full facilities.

:: Ratings

BEAUTY: ★ ★ ★ ★
PRIVACY: ★ ★ ★
SPACIOUSNESS: ★ ★ ★ ★
QUIET: ★ ★ ★ ★
SECURITY: ★ ★ ★ ★ ★
CLEANLINESS: ★ ★ ★ ★

The campground is fitted with old-fashioned fire rings of stone that have been cemented together for that rustic look and have a small round grate that is vertically adjustable for cooking. The paved pull-ins and campground roads cut down on the dust. The road splits and the electric sites end, keeping the RVs in their own part of the campground. A small stream bisects the campground.

The outer road has 21 of the best tent sites. They are deepest into the woods and farthest from the action. The inner road has 10 nice campsites, but they have campers on both sides of them. However, all the sites in the campground have adequate site privacy and spaciousness.

Both electric and nonelectric sites can be reserved. Only 10 sites are available on a first come, first served basis. Make reservations if you are coming here on a summer weekend or holiday, and ask for any site numbered 15 to 22. These are my favorites. Repeat campers often find a favorite site and stick with it. Be apprised that double campsites, with larger accommodations, cost a bit more.

It's hard to add to the beauty of an area such as this, but I have to hand it to the forest service. Rockcliff Lake is pretty. This 17-acre man-made body of water attracts swimmers and anglers alike. The white sandy beach looked like a good swimming launch, but the weather was a little too cool

:: Key Information

ADDRESS: Trout Pond Recreation Area, 814 Trout Pond Campground Road, Lost City, WV 26810

OPERATED BY: U.S. Forest Service

CONTACT: 540-984-4101, **www.fs.usda .gov/gwj;** reservations 877-444-6777, **reserveamerica.com**

OPEN: May–November

SITES: 11 electric, 25 nonelectric

SITE AMENITIES: Picnic table, fire ring, lantern post, tent pad

ASSIGNMENT: First come, first served unless reserved

REGISTRATION: Online, by phone, or at entrance booth

FACILITIES: Warm showers, flush toilets, water spigots

PARKING: At campsites only

FEE: May–Aug.: $19 per night nonelectric, $22 electric; Aug.–Nov.: $15 per night nonelectric, $18 electric

ELEVATION: 2,100 feet

RESTRICTIONS:
- **Pets:** On leash only
- **Fires:** In fire rings only
- **Alcohol:** At campsites only
- **Vehicles:** None
- **Boats:** No gas motors
- **Other:** 14-day stay limit

for me that day. Folks were fishing for trout. No gas motors are allowed on the lake, making for a peaceful setting. Nearby Trout Pond also has trout (imagine that). There is a limit of four fish per day.

A trail leads from the campground to Trout Pond and continues to Rockcliff Lake. The Rockcliff Lake Trail makes a 1-mile loop around the impoundment, passing rock outcrops and going over the dam. For a short geology lesson, take the Trout Pond Trail; it leaves right from the campground. Go left from the campground to see some of the sinkholes and depressions that are common in the area. You can make about a 2.5-mile loop by turning left on the Chimney Rock Trail and returning to the campground via Rockcliff Lake.

More ambitious hikers can make a 7-mile loop. Go right on Trout Pond Trail and turn left at Road 59, then left again on the Long Mountain Trail, then left again to intersect the far side of the Trout Pond Trail. Get a Trout Pond Recreation Area map from the forest service or the campground hosts, who look out for things during spring and summer.

Before you arrive, get supplies. There are none available nearby. Besides, once here, why leave until you have had your fill of the campground by West Virginia's only natural lake?

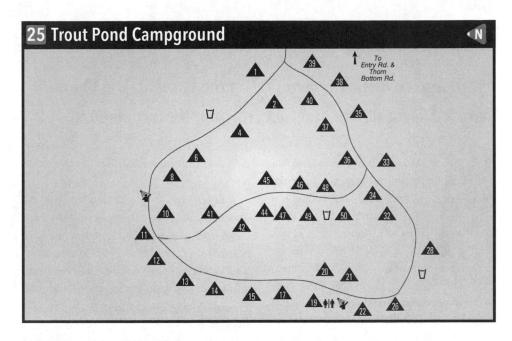

:: Getting There

From Wardensville, drive south on WV 259 for 18 miles to the hamlet of Lost River. Turn left on Mill Gap/Thorn Bottom Road (CR 16), and follow it 5 miles to FR 500. Turn right on FR 500 and follow it 1.7 miles to the gate of Trout Pond Recreation Area.

GPS COORDINATES   N38° 57.351′   W78° 44.154′

26

Wolf Gap

Wolf Gap is a rustic campground on the Virginia–West Virginia border. Hike state line trails directly from the campground.

We **all** know that West Virginia was once part of old Virginia. I am glad that the state line is where it is, making Wolf Gap a part of West Virginia. That way I could enjoy a stay here and include it in this book. And it is barely in West Virginia. You can actually throw a rock into the Old Dominion from a few of the campsites here. This campground is located in a gap along Old North Mountain, a long, northeast-southwest ridge over which the state line runs. Scenic high-country trails head in both directions through this section of the George Washington National Forest. And what better place to camp than Wolf Gap, where these trails are but footsteps away?

The campground is located in a transitional forest. Hickory, oak, and dogwood trees, more characteristic of the lower ridges and southern forests, are found here. Also here are birch and cherry, more typical of northern hardwood forests. How appropriate that these trees come together in an area that was literally divided by war between the North and South. There is also some white pine and a steady understory of cherry and maple.

Enter Wolf Gap and turn left into the campground. It is a small loop that rises away from the gap. The first few sites are flat, but then a little landscaping and leveling had to be done to make the other sites habitable. Campsites 2, 3, and 4 overlook Virginia. You will probably be gathering firewood in that state.

Most of the sites are on the outside of the loop. The layout has been tastefully done with stonework. You may have to walk up or down a few stone steps to reach your picnic table or tent pad. The sites are average-to-big in size and are well spaced from one another. With only 10 sites, you won't feel cramped. It can fill on weekends, but take a chance here. During the week it can get lonely at Wolf Gap. I know—I camped here on a Monday by myself. Also, notice there are no trash cans here. This is a "pack it in, pack it out" campground.

Campsites 7 and 8 are the best. They are highest on the hill and are the most spacious and private. Pass the Mill Mountain trailhead, and then come to the final two campsites that look toward West Virginia. They also are among the best. In the center of the loop are new-design vault toilets, using SST (Sweet-Smelling Technology). They are an improvement over the hole-in-the-ground-with-a-shed-over-it models of yesteryear. Trust me on this one. Over toward Wolf Gap

:: Ratings

BEAUTY: ★ ★ ★
PRIVACY: ★ ★ ★
SPACIOUSNESS: ★ ★ ★ ★
QUIET: ★ ★ ★ ★ ★
SECURITY: ★ ★ ★
CLEANLINESS: ★ ★ ★

:: Key Information

ADDRESS: Wolf Gap Campground, 109 Molineau Road, Edinburgh, VA 22834

OPERATED BY: U.S. Forest Service

CONTACT: 540-984-4101, www.fs.usda.gov/gwj

OPEN: Year-round

SITES: 10

SITE AMENITIES: Picnic table, fire ring, lantern post, tent pad

ASSIGNMENT: First come, first served; no reservations

REGISTRATION: Self-registration on-site

FACILITIES: Pump well, vault toilets

PARKING: At campsites only

FEE: None

ELEVATION: 2,600 feet

RESTRICTIONS:

■ **Pets:** On leash only

■ **Fires:** In fire rings only

■ **Alcohol:** At campsites only

■ **Vehicles:** None

■ **Other:** 14-day stay limit

is an attractive picnic area with a level lawn. The working hand-pump well is over here, but the water was too rusty for me to drink. Bring your own water to be on the safe side. What is a couple of bucks for water when you can camp here for free?

So what about the trails? On the campground side of the gap, the Mill Mountain Trail heads north. Mill Mountain is a knob on Great North Mountain. But before Mill Mountain is a superb rock lookout called Big Schloss. Head up the Mill Mountain Trail 2 miles, and take the 0.3-mile trail to the Big Schloss. German settlers on the Virginia side of the mountain called it the Castle— "schloss" means castle in German. Or maybe it means fantastic lookout over Massanutten Mountain and the Shenandoah Valley in Virginia and views into West Virginia. This

is a must for Wolf Gap campers. You can keep going on the Mill Mountain Trail and come to Sandstone Spring at 4.5 miles. The water is not rusty there.

On the south side of the gap is the Tibbet Knob Trail. It is a shorter but steeper walk to the top of Tibbet Knob. The trail then swings almost north again, following the state line, and heads toward Devils Hole Mountain. More good views can be had from Half Moon Mountain Trail. Drive 5 miles down into West Virginia from Wolf Gap and look for the hiker sign on your right. This is the Half Moon Trail. Cross Trout Run and walk 2.6 miles to the Half Moon Lookout Trail. Turn left on the Half Moon Lookout Trail, and follow it 0.8 mile to a rock lookout over Trout Run Valley. Get used to it; you'll be looking down on everyone while at Wolf Gap.

26 Wolf Gap Campground

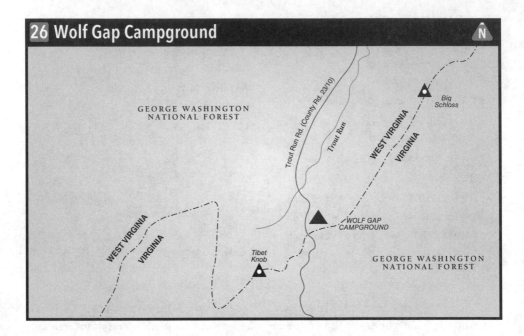

:: Getting There

From Wardensville, drive south on Trout Run Road (CR 23/10) for 13.5 miles to Wolf Gap at the state line. The campground will be on your left.

GPS COORDINATES   N38° 55.427′   W78° 41.374′

Feudin'
Country

27

Beech Fork State Park

Beech Fork has the largest campground in the state park system. And there is more than the lakeside setting to draw visitors.

This is an old-fashioned state park that serves recreationists of many stripes from the Huntington area and beyond. Beech Fork combines natural pleasures, such as hiking and nature programs, with organized outdoor activities, such as volleyball and basketball. Add water pursuits, such as fishing and boating, and mix in a swimming pool and the state park system's largest campground, and you get Beech Fork State Park.

Beech Fork Campground is big, really big. It was built by the Army Corps of Engineers right on the shore of Beech Fork Lake. The setting allows you to enjoy the lake and the hills, which rise out of the watershed. However, the campground itself is on an artificial flat created by the Corps of Engineers.

Pass the park office and come first to the Old Orchard Camping Area. It is open year-round and has water, sewer, and electrical hookups. The sites are crammed together and look like a parking lot. And it is—for RVs. Do not stay here.

:: Ratings

BEAUTY: ★ ★ ★
PRIVACY: ★ ★ ★
SPACIOUSNESS: ★ ★ ★ ★ ★
QUIET: ★ ★ ★ ★
SECURITY: ★ ★ ★ ★ ★
CLEANLINESS: ★ ★ ★ ★ ★

Turn left and cross a bridge over upper Beech Fork, just where the stream flows into the lake. This is the Moxley Branch Camping Area. Its campsites are strung out in various loops and spurs, with many along the lake. The landscape is mainly grass, with some planted trees getting big enough to provide shade. There is one bathhouse and a restroom for the loop. These campsites can be reserved, and you might want to reserve a site here on a busy holiday.

Back out on the main road, the Four Coves Camping Area has 88 sites and a bathhouse. Four peninsulas jut out between watery coves that make for an attractive setting. Many trees scattered about are awash in a grassy lawn. Most campsites lie along the water. Many campers pull their boats right up to their campsites.

Pass the boat launch area and come to the final camping area, the Lakeview Camping Area. Four spur roads end in loops with numerous waterside sites and good views of the lake. There is a bathhouse here too. Overall, the campground is spread out enough to make it seem smaller than it really is. It is aesthetically pleasing. The campsites are very spacious, but most are a little on the open side, which I personally don't like. So you might as well get friendly with your neighbor.

At Beech Fork, the campground is not the be all and end all. It is what you do with your time that counts. There are many

:: Key Information

ADDRESS: Beech Fork State Park, 5601 Long Branch Road, Barboursville, WV 25504

OPERATED BY: West Virginia State Parks

CONTACT: 304-528-5794, beechforksp.com; reservations at reservationfriend.com

OPEN: Old Orchard Camping Area: year-round; rest of campground: April 15–October 31

SITES: 49 full hookups, 226 electric

SITE AMENITIES: Picnic table, fire grate

ASSIGNMENT: Reservations accepted but not required

REGISTRATION: Online, by phone, or ranger will come by

FACILITIES: Hot showers, flush toilets, water spigots, coin laundry, camp store in summer

PARKING: At campsites only

FEE: $33 per night full hookup, $28 electric, $24 nonelectric

ELEVATION: 600 feet

RESTRICTIONS:

■ **Pets:** On leash only

■ **Fires:** In fire grates only

■ **Alcohol:** Prohibited

■ **Vehicles:** None

■ **Other:** 14-day stay limit

hiking trails, from the 0.75-mile Nature Trail to the 5-mile Lost Trail that is open to hikers and mountain bikers. The Lakeview Trail passes an old log cabin and pioneer cemetery. The Fitness Trail has exercise stations for those inclined to challenge more than their legs and lungs.

The lake draws many boaters and anglers casting for tiger muskie, saugeye, bluegill, catfish, and bass. There is a 10-horsepower motor limit on the lake and many no-wake areas, such as around the campground. Rowboats and paddleboats are rented in summer. The fishing here is good from the bank too.

This park comes alive in summer. Ranger-led interpretive programs help you enjoy the natural aspects of the park, and there are also sporting venues for volleyball, tennis, basketball, horseshoes, and baseball or softball.

If it is really hot, you can cool off in the park pool. Swimming is not allowed in the lake. You can check out the game room on a rainy day. Though supplies are available in Huntington, there is a camp store open in the summer. If you can't find anything to do here at Beech Fork State Park, you might as well get back to the couch and click the remote.

27 Beech Fork State Park Campground

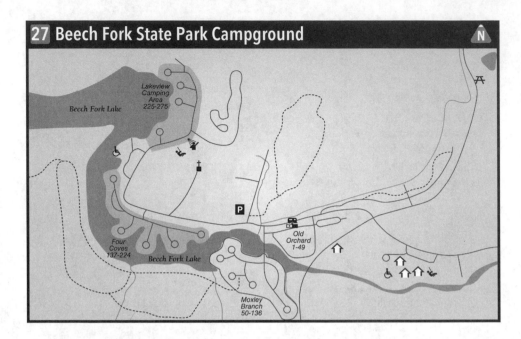

:: Getting There

From I-64 near Huntington, take Exit 11 and head south on WV 10. Follow WV 10 for 1.5 miles to Green Valley Road. Turn right on Green Valley Road and follow it for 7 miles to the state park, which will be on your right.

GPS COORDINATES   N38° 18.487'   W82° 20.879'

Cabwaylingo State Forest

Campers can enjoy two campgrounds in a forest with the stonework of the Depression-era Civilian Conservation Corps.

The name Cabwaylingo is the combination of the counties of which it is a part: Cabell, Wayne, Lincoln, and Mingo. But what's in a name? In this case, you get two neat campgrounds that offer different experiences and a lot of rugged terrain.

West Virginia saw this as a good candidate for a state forest back in the 1930s, as it was one of the original state forests. During the Great Depression, the Civilian Conservation Corps developed the forest—not too much, but just enough to make it feel homey. Their stone handiwork and the Tick Ridge Campground hearken back to the old days of camping, when tent camping was the only way to do it. The CCC also built trails that we can walk today.

But there is also a newer side to the Cabwaylingo, such as the pool for hot summer days and the 11-site Spruce Creek Campground, which has many modern features. Built along Spruce Creek, this camping area offers three campsites spread along the creek with water and electricity—which spells RVs. The bathhouse is here. Across

the bridge over Spruce Creek are three more RV sites, but off to the right are five tent-only sites that have electricity. Steep ridges give the campground a closed-in feel. Partway up these ridges near the campground entrance are two CCC-built stone shelters that are a real treat to see.

The other campground, Tick Ridge, is a throwback to the days of yesteryear. A gravel road leads from the park's main waterway, Twelvepole Creek, up to the top of Tick Ridge. Just past the road toward Marcum Cemetery is the first camping loop. This loop is in a pine/oak forest with six campsites. All but one of the campsites are on the inside of the loop. The understory is minimal and the woods drop off steeply on all sides. The bathhouse and a water spigot are adjacent to this loop. The grills and a picnic shelter are CCC stonework.

Three campsites continue along the narrow neck of the ridge before it widens out. The final loop is perched on the mountainside, where the only level spots are where you pitch your tent and use your picnic table. All around are great views deep into the forest of oak, tulip trees, and more. Some sites have been allowed to revert to the forest. Pass the Indian Trail, and the spread-out campground continues, with private sites set all along Tick Ridge at different elevations and perspectives. Pit toilets and water spigots are conveniently spread around. It's a safe bet that you will

:: Ratings

BEAUTY: ★ ★ ★ ★
PRIVACY: ★ ★ ★
SPACIOUSNESS: ★ ★ ★
QUIET: ★ ★ ★ ★
SECURITY: ★ ★ ★ ★ ★
CLEANLINESS: ★ ★ ★ ★

:: Key Information

ADDRESS: Cabwaylingo State Forest, Route 1, Box 85, Dunlow, WV 25511

OPERATED BY: West Virginia State Parks

CONTACT: 304-385-4255; cabwaylingo.com

OPEN: April–October

SITES: Tick Ridge, 10; Spruce Creek, 11

SITE AMENITIES: Tick Ridge: picnic table, fire grate; Spruce Creek: electricity, water, picnic table, fire grate

ASSIGNMENT: First come, first served; no reservations

REGISTRATION: Ranger will come by

FACILITIES: Tick Ridge: showers, water spigots, vault toilets; Spruce Creek: hot showers, flush toilets

PARKING: At campsites only

FEE: Spruce Creek, $20 or 26 per night; Tick Ridge, $12

ELEVATION: Tick Ridge, 1,300 feet; Spruce Creek, 800 feet

RESTRICTIONS:
- **Pets:** On leash only
- **Fires:** In fire grates only
- **Alcohol:** Prohibited
- **Vehicles:** None
- **Other:** 14-day stay limit

get a campsite here, even on weekends. This campground fills only during major summer holidays.

There are nearly 25 miles of trails to trek. The Indian Trail leaves the campground and leads a mile down toward the park's group camp. Just a short distance from Tick Ridge is the CCC-built fire tower. You can no longer climb the 1934-era tower itself, but just a few hundred yards of walking takes you from Tick Ridge to obscured views at the tower base. For rock formations, take the Copley Trail. Use the Sleepy Hollow and Martin Ridge Trails for a 3.5-mile partial loop, which you could complete with a bit of road-walking along Twelvepole Creek.

The creek is stocked with trout during the spring months. Watch for the waterfall along Sleepy Hollow Trail.

Near Spruce Creek Campground is the Beech Ridge Trail. Take this trail up to Tick Ridge Road, and then loop back down Spruce Creek Trail to the campground. Get a trail map from the park office, and lace up your shoes.

The basketball court can provide a good diversion. You may want to cool off in the park swimming pool, which is open Memorial Day–Labor Day. This place is mostly about relaxation and getting back to nature. And that is an important part of any tent-camping experience.

28 Cabwaylingo State Forest: Spruce Creek Campground

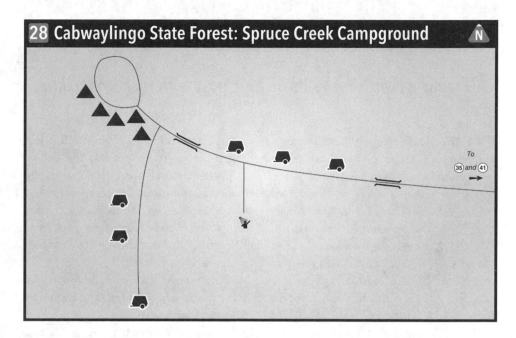

:: Getting There

From Huntington, drive south on WV 152 for about 42 miles; then turn left on Missouri Branch Road (CR 35), and you'll soon come to the state forest.

GPS COORDINATES   N37° 58.123′   W82° 21.353′

29

Chief Logan State Park

This state park integrates its historic past with modern facilities.

Southern West Virginia has historically been coal country, with some of the most extensive seams in the United States. Before the arrival of white settlers, Mingo Indians called this area home. Chief Logan State Park, the recreational heart of this rich land, is named after the most renowned Mingo, Chief Logan. The parkland was once part of Merrill Coal Company. Now, this area of wooded hills, cut with deep hollows of the Buffalo Creek watershed, is well developed with an eye toward local recreationists, yet it stays true to its past, with historical exhibits and more highlighting the American Indian, settler, and coal era of times gone by.

The campground is adequate for the park, which has much to see and do. You can hike its trails, swim in the pool, play on the game courts, go horseback riding, or see the wildlife exhibit. And during parts of the summer, you can see *The Aracoma Story*, a play about the era when the Mingo first encountered British settlers exploring the continent.

To find the campground, drive past the park restaurant, which serves hungry campers good meals, and turn left along Buffalo Creek. At the head of the hollow is the campground. First, pass many fully equipped pull-through campsites that attract the big rigs. These line the main road. Cross over Buffalo Creek, and more fully equipped sites continue. The modern bathhouse is on your left.

Finally, arrive at a turn to your right. Veer up the hill to a bench where five campsites spoke out from a small loop. These overlook the hollow. Grass borders the tables and grates. There is some shade and no RVs.

There is another appealing camping area at the very head of the hollow. There, five sites have paved pull-in areas, as do all the camp-sites. Some of the sites are in full sun, but chances are you can get whatever campsite pleases you because the tent sites never fill. Most park visitors are locals who just come for the day. This leaves visitors from outside the area to enjoy the camping pleasures along with the park's recreation activities.

Your first order of business is to gain insight into the area's history. From the campground, take the Coal Mine Trail. This path traces an old mine tram road past mine openings and a tipple site. You can also see a coal silo. The trail is a mile long and a good leg stretcher. Next, drive down and look at the pioneer homestead and the locomotive on display. The homestead will make you appreciate modern conveniences. Steam locomotives, such as the one here, were essential in moving coal from the point of extraction to market.

:: Ratings

BEAUTY: ★ ★ ★
PRIVACY: ★ ★ ★
SPACIOUSNESS: ★ ★ ★
QUIET: ★ ★ ★ ★
SECURITY: ★ ★ ★ ★ ★
CLEANLINESS: ★ ★ ★ ★

:: Key Information

ADDRESS: Chief Logan State Park, Logan, WV 25601

OPERATED BY: West Virginia State Parks

CONTACT: 304-792-7125, chiefloganstatepark.com

OPEN: March–November

SITES: 14 water, sewer, and electric; 12 water and electric only

SITE AMENITIES: Picnic table, fire grate

ASSIGNMENT: Reservations accepted but not required

REGISTRATION: Ranger will come by to register you

FACILITIES: Hot showers, flush toilets, water spigot

PARKING: At campsites only

FEE: $27 per night

ELEVATION: 1,500 feet

RESTRICTIONS:

■ **Pets:** On leash only

■ **Fires:** In fire grates only

■ **Alcohol:** Prohibited

■ **Vehicles:** None

■ **Other:** 14-day stay limit

Learn about the natural history of the area either on other park trails or at the wildlife exhibit. The wildlife exhibit features native flora and fauna like birds, boars, bears, and snakes. Here, you can learn from a park naturalist about the daily life of local woodland creatures.

Hikers and mountain bikers can explore some of the park's 3,300 acres via 18 miles of trails. The Woodpecker Trail winds up the hollow of Buffalo Creek. The Guyandotte Beauty Trail is great for wildflowers in the spring and passes more mining ruins. Of special note is the Fitness Trail, which has exercise stations along the way.

After your hike, cool off at the park pool. This watery getaway spells relaxation. Hills rise from either side of the swimming area. The game courts and miniature golf course are located here too. Playgrounds are scattered throughout the park.

There is a Civil War Reenactment at the park toward the end of September. Summer weekends feature plays put on at the outdoor theater. *The Aracoma Story* is an annual draw that features the compelling story of the ill-fated love between a chief's daughter and a British soldier. The setting accentuates the story. The setting at Chief Logan State Park will accentuate your tent camping experience too.

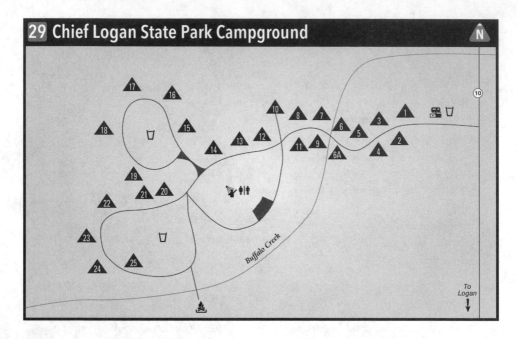

:: Getting There

From the town of Logan, head north on WV 10 for 4 miles. Chief Logan State Park will be on your left.

GPS COORDINATES   N37° 53.145'   W82° 01.856'

30

Guyandotte

This Army Corps of Engineers lake is one of southern West Virginia's recreational secrets.

The Army Corps of Engineers has built many dams across our nation. Most of these have been built for flood control, as is the case at R.D. Bailey Lake. Recreation is secondary and thus has not been promoted. The end result is flood control for the Guyandotte River Valley and a little-used recreation area that is a hidden gem of coal country. The attractive campground is large, and an open campsite is guaranteed. This way, you can focus on enjoying the scenic lake tucked away in the mountains of Wyoming and Mingo Counties.

I enjoyed a personal tour of the area by a park staffer. You could sense the pride in his voice as we checked out the facilities. After enjoying the view from the visitor center (a must), we drove to the Guyandotte Campground. The entrance road to the campground traces an old railroad grade along the Guyandotte River.

The campground is broken into four sections strung out along the river valley. Each area has its own self-registration station. Cross the old railroad bridge and come to the Reedy Creek area. It has 31 campsites set along an oval loop. The riverside terrain is heavily wooded, with thick brush offering campsite privacy. Five campsites offer direct access to the Guyandotte River. All the campsites have paved pull-ins. The fully equipped bathhouse is in the center of the oval.

The Locust Branch area has 62 campsites, 13 of which offer river access. It is the most popular loop. These riverside campsites are heavily wooded and spread far apart. The upper area, set away from the water, is more open and hilly. There is a variety of shaded or open campsites. The camping areas up here are a little on the small side but have been leveled for ease of setting up your tent. A bathhouse and the campground pay phone are located on this loop.

The Guyandotte River continues its sharp bend curving along the Sugarcamp Branch camping area. Eleven of the 55 sites here are riverside but are open to the sun and to other campers because they are too close together. These are the least desirable river-access sites. The upper area has hillside campsites, some of which are pull-through. There are all varieties of sun and shade, but generally the campsites are a little too close together.

The Smith Bend area has 17 campsites, none of which access the Guyandotte. A bathhouse and picnic shelter are on this

:: Ratings

BEAUTY: ★ ★ ★
PRIVACY: ★ ★ ★ ★
SPACIOUSNESS: ★ ★ ★
QUIET: ★ ★ ★ ★ ★
SECURITY: ★ ★ ★ ★
CLEANLINESS: ★ ★ ★ ★ ★

:: Key Information

ADDRESS: R.D. Bailey Lake, P.O. Drawer 70, Justice, WV 24851

OPERATED BY: Army Corps of Engineers

CONTACT: 304-664-3220, **www.lrh .usace.army.mil/missions/recreation /westvirginia/rdbaileylake.aspx**

OPEN: Memorial Day–Labor Day

SITES: 5 primitive, 163 electric

SITE AMENITIES: Picnic table, fire grate, electricity

ASSIGNMENT: First come, first served; no reservations

REGISTRATION: Self-registration on-site

FACILITIES: Hot showers, flush toilets, water spigots, pay phone

PARKING: At campsites only

FEE: $16 electric

ELEVATION: 1,040 feet

RESTRICTIONS:

- **Pets:** On leash only
- **Fires:** In fire grates only
- **Alcohol:** Prohibited
- **Vehicles:** None
- **Other:** 3 cars and 8 campers per site

two-way road. Fewer campsites and proximity to the boat ramp are its best features.

Reedy Creek is my favorite camping locale. The Sugarcamp and Smith Bend areas may not be open until the other areas begin to fill. There are always campsites available, even on summer holiday weekends. One interesting aspect of the campground is your departure route. It passes through an old railroad tunnel on the way back to the main road.

Each loop has horseshoe pits and a playground area for kids. Cyclists will enjoy the quiet paved roads of the large campground. There are volleyball and basketball courts near the campground boat ramp.

Most recreation, however, centers on the lake. And a scenic lake it is: cliffs line the dammed section of the Guyandotte that snakes toward the impressive dam. Swimmers enjoy both the lake and the river. Ski boats and personal watercraft tour the narrow impoundment. If you don't have a boat, they are available at the Guyandotte Point Boat Ramp and Marina. Anglers vie for bass, bream, crappie, and catfish on the banks or by boat.

The main purpose of the $180 million R.D. Bailey project is flood control. The Guyandotte River used to overflow about every other year. It has been under control since 1980, when the 13-year project was finished. To learn more, check out the dam tours led by Corps personnel. To tour the dam, leave the campground and return to WV 97. Turn right on WV 97 and follow it 2.2 miles to US 52. Turn right on US 52 and follow it 1.1 miles to the right turn into the Visitor Center.

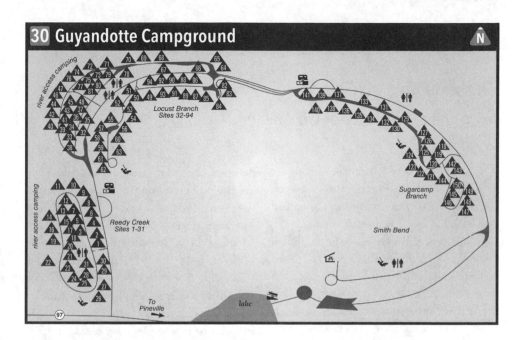

:: Getting There

From Pineville, drive west on WV 97 for 18 miles to a paved road where there is a large sign for the Guyandotte Campground. Turn right onto the paved road, pass the guard station, and drive 5.8 miles to the campground.

GPS COORDINATES   N37° 36.709'   W81° 44.472'

31

Kanawha State Forest

This mountain getaway is only 7 miles but feels a world away from the capital city of Charleston.

Kanawha State Forest has been under state control for more than seven decades. The city of Charleston has spread to Kanawha, and that growth has made the natural world of Kanawha that much more valuable. When you are back here, it is hard to believe the gold capitol dome is just a few ridges away. The Davis Creek Camping Area has a rustic aura, and some park facilities, built by the Civilian Conservation Corps, add an old-timey touch. But the daily drawing cards are the trails that bring mountain bikers, hikers, and horseback riders to comb the hills and valleys of the Kanawha.

The Davis Creek Camping Area has a different twist. Most campgrounds start at the bottom of a valley and work their way up, then turn around. This campground starts at the top of the hollow, works its way down, then turns around.

Enter the upper end of Davis Creek, which is just a small stream at this point, and begin to pass the first campsites to your right. These first sites are rustic and strung along the creek with plenty of distance between them for adequate privacy. They are equipped with only a picnic table and a fire pit made of local stone. One of the first seven campsites is directly creekside. All are adequately level beneath the riparian forest of beech and sycamore, with steep, wooded hills rising from the creek's edge. Look for the hornbeam tree, also known as muscle-wood, with its sinewy trunks that resemble a human arm or leg. It grows beside streams and in ravines in mountainous terrain.

Cross a bridge over Davis Creek, and seven rustic campsites are situated on a side hollow and stream. Pass the bathhouse just before you turn left into this hollow. Hemlocks shade some of the campsites, and the smallish valley seems even more intimate.

Back on the main road, a cluster of good tent sites abuts Davis Creek. Cross a small footbridge to get to campsite 21. After this, all the sites are equipped with water and electricity, but, ironically, most are less level than the rustic campsites. Below you, on a one-way return road, are four campsites in small flats that are the best and the most private in the campground. Davis Hollow is not big-rig-friendly. Overall, none of the campsites are too big, but you can find privacy.

Come to the second bathhouse farther down the long hollow, and cross yet another bridge. Some sites are along the creek and others are on the hillside. They are well spread apart. The paved road loops around. A short gravel spur goes a bit farther down

:: Ratings

BEAUTY: ★ ★ ★ ★
PRIVACY: ★ ★ ★
SPACIOUSNESS: ★ ★ ★
QUIET: ★ ★ ★ ★
SECURITY: ★ ★ ★ ★ ★
CLEANLINESS: ★ ★ ★ ★ ★

:: Key Information

ADDRESS: Kanawha State Forest,
Route 2, Box 285,
Charleston, WV 25314

OPERATED BY: West Virginia State Parks

CONTACT: 304-558-3500,
kanawhastateforest.com

OPEN: Mid-April–early December

SITES: 21 nonelectric, 25 electric

SITE AMENITIES: Picnic table, fire pit

ASSIGNMENT: Reservations accepted
Memorial Day–Labor Day; otherwise
first come, first served

REGISTRATION: By phone, or ranger will
come by

FACILITIES: Hot showers, flush toilets,
coin laundry

PARKING: At campsites only

FEE: $20 per night nonelectric,
$26 electric

ELEVATION: 980 feet

RESTRICTIONS:

■ **Pets:** On leash only

■ **Fires:** In fire pits only

■ **Alcohol:** Prohibited

■ **Vehicles:** 30-foot trailer limit

■ **Other:** 14-day stay limit

the creek and has larger sites designed for trailers under the 30-foot length limit, though I wouldn't want to drive one back this way.

The campground fills only on the three major summer holidays: Memorial Day, Independence Day, and Labor Day. Mountain bikers and hikers love this place. Kanawha is laced with trails that course through more than 11,000 acres of preserved terrain. There are even some stands of old-growth forest in Kanawha among the 25-plus miles of trails. You can try out the Store Hollow and Davis Creek Trails from the campground. Mountain bikers really take to the Davis Creek Trail that leaves the lower end of the campground. Take the Overlook Rock Trail for a view and the Hemlock Falls Trail for some water. Many of the trails are hiking only. Stop in the park office and get a good trail map; then set out on your own jaunt.

You may want to ride a horse. The D&M Stables are located right in the forest and offer one- and two-hour trail rides for a fee. A good family activity is their horse-drawn hayride. The pond near the park entrance, built by the CCC, is stocked with bass and bluegill for anglers. Everyone comes to relax in the campground, but many locals like to recline poolside at the forest swimming pool. Kids love the pool and the playground. There's a little bit for everybody at this woodland getaway in the mountains a short drive from the state capital.

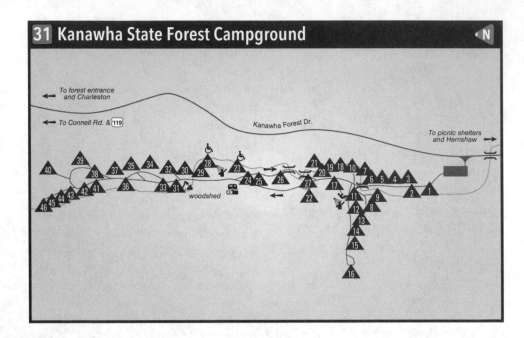

:: Getting There

From I-64 in Charleston, take Exit 58A, and drive south on US 119. Turn left onto Oakwood Road at the second stoplight. Turn right onto Bridge Road, then right onto Connell Road. At the bottom of Connell Road, make a sharp left on Kanawha Forest Drive and follow it to the forest entrance. Brown state forest signs will guide you from US 119.

GPS COORDINATES   N38° 16.886′   W81° 38.518′

32

Panther WMA

Visit the hills and hollows of West Virginia's deep south.

Panther WMA is located near the intersection of Virginia, Kentucky, and West Virginia and is the southernmost campground described in this guidebook. This region, steeped in coal-mining culture, is characterized by deep and narrow hollows with swift creeks at the bottom and hills rising above. These hills make up in steepness what they lack in height, compared to more lofty places in the Mountain State. A small, quiet, and never-filled campground is located in one of the few level locales in the area. From here, you can enjoy many of the natural and man-made features that Panther WMA offers.

The campground is located at the confluence of Panther Creek and Crane Branch in a wooded flat. The six campsites are strung out next to Panther Creek. Overhead, a forest of beech, hemlock, sycamore, and yellow birch provides seasonal shade. The understory is mossy beneath the trees and grassy in adjacent open areas.

Campsite 1 overlooks Crane Branch emptying into Panther Creek. It has an old-fashioned fire pit built of stone and concrete. This campsite is one of the two most popular sites, at a campground that doesn't fill even on July 4. Walk the footbridge over Crane Branch and come to campsite 2. It also has the old-style fire pit. Campsite 3 is the most open. It lies next to a grassy clearing but is short on flat tent sites. Campsite 4 is across the grassy clearing but also next to Panther Creek. Campsite 5 was my choice. It has the largest level area and is very close to Panther Creek. Campsite 6 lies beneath a huge beech tree and has disabled access. It is the only campsite that has a paved parking pull-in. This is the most popular campsite of them all.

A vault toilet and hand-pump well are located just across the forest road from the intimate campground. The odd thing about this campground is the electrical outlets for each site, a feature that's rarely combined with vault toilets and hand-pump wells. But no matter—the electricity will only be to your advantage and will not be much of an attraction to RVs, or anyone else, for that matter. You'll likely have this underused resource to yourself any day of the week.

I recommend coming in the spring because the wildflowers here are incredible. During my stay the trilliums, among many wildflowers, really put on a show. Inquire by phone about bloom times.

Hot showers are available at the bathhouse for the swimming pool. The pool, along with the children's wading pool, is a big family attraction and is open Memorial Day–Labor Day. There is also a playground

:: Ratings

BEAUTY: ★ ★ ★
PRIVACY: ★ ★ ★ ★
SPACIOUSNESS: ★ ★ ★ ★ ★
QUIET: ★ ★ ★ ★
SECURITY: ★ ★ ★
CLEANLINESS: ★ ★ ★ ★

:: Key Information

ADDRESS: Panther WMA,
Box 287, Panther, WV 24872

OPERATED BY: West Virginia State Parks

CONTACT: 304-938-2252,
pantherstateforest.com

OPEN: Mid-April–October

SITES: 6

SITE AMENITIES: Picnic table, fire grate,
electricity

ASSIGNMENT: First come, first served;
no reservations

REGISTRATION: Ranger will come by to
register you

FACILITIES: Pump well, vault toilet, electricity; showers available Memorial Day–
Labor Day

PARKING: At campsites only

FEE: $13 per night

ELEVATION: 985 feet

RESTRICTIONS:

- **Pets:** On leash only
- **Fires:** In fire grates only
- **Alcohol:** Prohibited
- **Vehicles:** None
- **Other:** 14-day stay limit

for kids to enjoy, along with several fine, developed picnic areas.

The rest of your activities will center around the natural amenities. With more than 22,000 acres, Panther WMA offers a lot of room to roam. Those adept with a rod and reel can ply the creeks. The waterways have smallmouth bass year-round and are stocked with trout March–May. Hikers can leave directly from the campground up the Crane Branch Trail to Buzzard Roost Over-look. Add the Loop Trail to this hike for a 2-mile round-trip. George's Fork Trail also leads to the Buzzard Roost. Drift Branch Trail leads 1.5 miles to the forest fire tower at

2,100 feet and views into three states. Twin Rocks Trail breaks off from the Drift Branch Trail and leads along Panther Creek toward the forest group camp.

There are many gas wells in Panther WMA. What this means for you is more than 15 miles of gated roads that offer more terrain to cover, whether you are on foot or a mountain bike. Get a trail map from the for-est headquarters before you come, but, by all means, come. Check ahead for hunting schedules if you plan to do some fall hiking or shooting. Also, acquire all your supplies before you get here, as there are no grocery stores or mega stores in the vicinity.

32 Panther WMA Campground

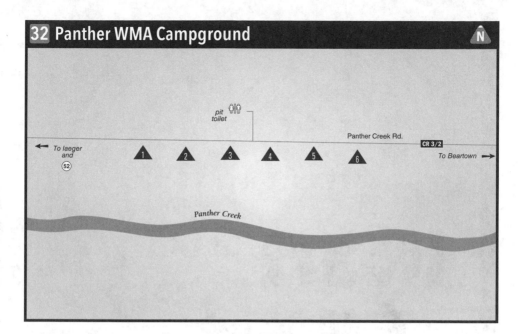

:: Getting There

From Iaeger, drive north on US 52 for 1 mile. Turn left on Route 3 at the forest sign to Panther. Continue 6 miles to the hamlet of Panther. Turn left at the Panther Post Office on CR 3/1, where the road splits into CR 3/2, and follow CR 3/2 for 3.5 miles to the forest entrance. The campground will be ahead on your right.

GPS COORDINATES   N37° 25.509′   W81° 51.656′

Heart
of West
Virginia

33

Audra State Park

This may be the prettiest campground in the state.

If I had all the elements of nature at my disposal and I were going to design a campground, I don't know if it would turn out any better than the campground at Audra State Park. Many times a campground will be attractive yet have some flaw that keeps it from being exceptional. This campground has no such flaws. It is exceptional. Why? The place is simply beautiful. Moreover, its design integrates man-made additions into the landscape, and it isn't overdeveloped.

Be forewarned: the campground is the attraction at Audra State Park. As you will see, the park setting is exceptionally scenic, but it is a small state park. What it does offer is A+ scenery: the aquamarine Middle Fork River rushing over rocks, the deep shady woods, thickets of rhododendron, precipitous hillsides littered with boulders. There are a few ways to enjoy this natural splendor, and there are some attractions in the area, but like others who return to Audra year after year, you come here to camp.

Drop steeply off the main park road and enter the campground, which is situated in a flat along the Middle Fork River, off to your right. Trees tower overhead. The river

:: Ratings

> BEAUTY: ★ ★ ★ ★ ★
> PRIVACY: ★ ★ ★ ★
> SPACIOUSNESS: ★ ★ ★
> QUIET: ★ ★ ★ ★ ★
> SECURITY: ★ ★ ★
> CLEANLINESS: ★ ★ ★ ★

noisily cascades in the distance. Make your way past the little-used campground check-in station, and you already see why this place is so great. Immense thickets of rhododendron intermingle with large boulders in a dense forest of hemlock. Campsites are tucked into small clearings that offer maximum camper privacy. On the outside of the loop, campsites lie next to the Middle Fork River. Many directly overlook and access the scenic waterway.

One site has a little footbridge to allow campers closer access to the stream. Small hemlocks fight for sunlight below the taller trees, as the sun shines brightly on the river. The sites on the inside of the loop are even more secluded, to the point that you might overlook them if you are driving faster than 5 miles per hour. However, the first of two bathhouses is fairly easy to spot. A small playground is located by one of the bathhouses. Water spigots are spread throughout the area.

The second half of the campground has more hardwoods and riverside sites, and the campsites are a little larger. Some sites have small beach areas at the water's edge. As the loop swings away from the Middle Fork, many campsites abut a taller bluff up from the river. Cabin-size boulders function as campsite barriers. Rhododendron thickets resume. This shrub blooms around late June–early July and is a sight to see. The hillside campsites may not be as level as the riverside sites, but they are as scenic and usually have a level tent site.

:: Key Information

ADDRESS: Audra State Park, Route 4, Box 564, Buckhannon, WV 26201

OPERATED BY: West Virginia State Parks

CONTACT: 304-457-1162, audrastatepark.com

OPEN: Mid-April–mid-October

SITES: 67

SITE AMENITIES: Picnic table, fire grate, movable wooden bench

ASSIGNMENT: First come, first served; no reservations

REGISTRATION: Ranger will come by to register you

FACILITIES: Hot showers, flush toilets, coin laundry

PARKING: At campsites only

FEE: $20 per night

ELEVATION: 1,700 feet

RESTRICTIONS:

■ **Pets:** On leash only

■ **Fires:** In fire grates only

■ **Alcohol:** Prohibited

■ **Vehicles:** None

■ **Other:** 14-day stay limit

There is no easy way to get to Audra, and there is a slight risk of not securing a campsite. Audra fills on Memorial Day weekend and most weekends in July. Other than that, you should be fine. The park superintendent says the best time to come is September; the weather is still good and Audra begins to show her fall colors.

Audra is named after a town that once stood in the area. Little remains of the community; the area has returned to its natural fairness. They don't even need a swimming pool here. The park just laid out a concrete beach extending into the Middle Fork and used Mother Nature's swimming hole. It is open Memorial Day–Labor Day; swim at your own risk.

A tram road along the river, once used by loggers, is now used as the trail to Alum Cave. There is an overhanging bluff and other scenic overlooks. Continue past Alum Cave, and the trail makes a 2.7-mile loop back to the park's picnic area. Another trail, the Rock Cliff Trail, leaves the campground and climbs the bluffs behind the campsites.

Kids like to play in the Middle Fork right at the campground or tube from the campground downstream to the swimming beach. Spring brings kayakers testing their skills on the Middle Fork from Audra to the confluence with the Tygart Valley River, which then descends into a deep gorge.

Barbour County, home of Audra State Park, has some interesting features. Nearby are two historic covered bridges; one was built in 1852, the other in 1856. The town of Philippi, where the first land battle of the Civil War purportedly occurred, is the site of an annual Blue and Gray Reunion in early summer. There's a museum with Civil War memorabilia near the covered bridge in Philippi where you can also get supplies. It may be the only time you want to get away from the campground at Audra State Park.

33 Audra State Park Campground

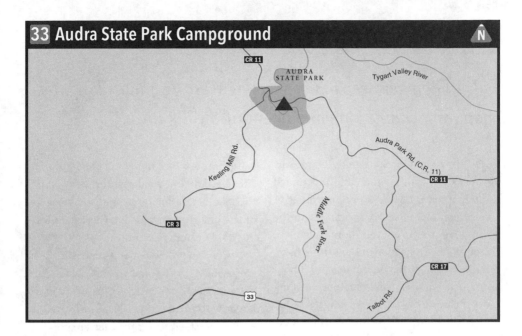

:: Getting There

From I-79 at Weston, take Exit 99 and follow US 33 east to Talbot Road. Turn left on Talbot Road and follow the signs to the state park.

GPS COORDINATES   N39° 02.299′   W80° 03.794′

34

Bakers Run

Bakers Run lies deep in the heart of West Virginia, along the mountain-rimmed impoundment of the Elk River.

What makes this campground worthy? It lies along an impounded stretch of the Elk River. It becomes a snake-like ribbon of still water, merging with the Holly River to make even more ribbons of water, collectively known as Sutton Lake, winding through the mountains. It is about fishing, swimming, and boating—whiling away the warm days of summer by the water.

Drop down into the river bottom where two camping areas are laid out. Pass the campground entrance station and turn right into the first camping area. This area, Mill Creek, does not have electric sites. Translation: no RVs. The campsites are laid out in two rows paralleling the shoreline. They are a little on the small side and don't have a whole lot of understory. Shade trees cover most of the campsites along the river.

The 14 lakeside campsites are the most desirable. The row away from the river is less shady and less desirable, though these campsites are closer to the fully equipped bathhouse, a playground, and a large field. Water spigots are evenly scattered about the

camping area. Five more well-shaded campsites lie along the road as it turns away from the lake. These sites are larger and are some of the first sites occupied in this much-less-busy, tent camper–friendly loop.

Continue down along the Elk River embayment, and come to the Bakers Run camping area on your right. This area is much larger, with 76 campsites. There are five tightly knit rows of electric sites that are so close together they look like an RV dealership. Do not camp here. However, 11 of these campsites are lakeside and will nearly always be taken.

The second half of the camping area is nonelectric and is much less crowded. This section, ironically, has more spacious campsites, though privacy is still minimal due to a lack of understory. Most of these sites are in the open, making for a summertime sun whipping. The saving grace of this area is the six mostly shaded campsites near the boat ramp. They have fantastic lake views. These campsites will be proudly scoffed up by most tent campers. The Bakers Run bathhouse is on a hill far above the campground.

The boat ramp at Bakers Run is one of your keys to enjoying Sutton Lake. Boating for pleasure is a big draw, with such lake and mountain scenery. You can cruise up the arm of the Holly River and to the marina at Gerald R. Freeman Recreation Area, or head downstream to the Sutton Dam and the Bee Run Recreation Area. Many side creeks also form slender arms for exploring. Most of

:: Ratings

BEAUTY: ★ ★ ★
PRIVACY: ★ ★ ★
SPACIOUSNESS: ★ ★ ★
QUIET: ★ ★ ★ ★ ★
SECURITY: ★ ★ ★ ★ ★
CLEANLINESS: ★ ★ ★ ★

:: Key Information

ADDRESS: Bakers Run Recreation Area, P.O. Box 426, Sutton, WV 26601

OPERATED BY: Army Corps of Engineers

CONTACT: 304-765-2816 or 304-765-5631, **www.lrh.usace.army.mil/missions/recreation/westvirginia/suttonlake.aspx**

OPEN: Late May–late October

SITES: 103 nonelectric, 27 electric

SITE AMENITIES: Picnic table, fire grate, lantern post

ASSIGNMENT: First come, first served; no reservations

REGISTRATION: At campground registration booth

FACILITIES: Hot showers, flush toilets, water spigots

PARKING: At campsites only

FEE: $16 per night nonelectric, $18–$24 electric (30 amp or 50 amp)

ELEVATION: 930 feet

RESTRICTIONS:

■ **Pets:** On leash only

■ **Fires:** In fire grates only

■ **Alcohol:** At campsites only

■ **Vehicles:** None

■ **Other:** 14-day stay limit in a 28-day period

these side creek embayments are no-wake zones so as not to disturb anglers and divers.

Anglers will be able to cast their lines for rainbow trout, walleye, bass, crappie, and catfish. The West Virginia Department of Natural Resources handles the fisheries here at Sutton Lake. If you don't have a boat, you can walk down to the Tunnel Road Fishing Access Area at the far end of Bakers Run.

In the campground, bikers can enjoy the quiet paved roads, though more ambitious riders can tool around on the gravel road that heads up Bakers Run. There is a basketball court and a horseshoe pit for game players. However, you are more likely to find relaxed campers who like to put a little water into their summertime camping adventures here at Sutton Lake.

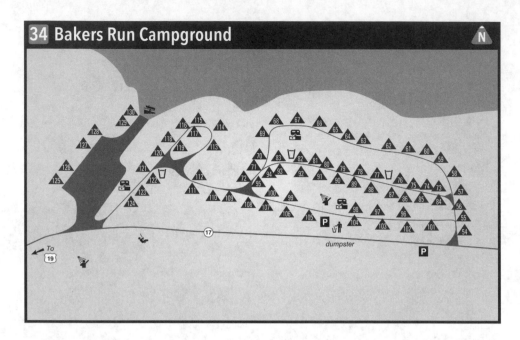

34 Bakers Run Campground

:: Getting There

From downtown Sutton, head south on old US 19 (CR 19/40) for 4.5 miles to WV 17 (Wolf Creek/Centralia Road). Turn left on WV 17 and follow it 10 miles to Bakers Run Recreation Area, which will be on your left.

GPS COORDINATES   N38° 38.123′   W80° 34.619′

35

Bulltown

Bulltown is set in a historic locale yet features many modern recreational facilities.

The **Bulltown** area has been busy through the centuries. It was once an American Indian stronghold. Later, settlers came in, building a mill on nearby Falls Creek to grind their corn. One of the few passable roads of the 1800s, the Weston and Gauley Turnpike, went through here. This strategic road was the site of a Civil War battle. Today, Bulltown is the site of an Army Corps of Engineers campground that is adjacent to Burnsville Lake, which backs up to a portion of the Little Kanawha River. The Bulltown Historical Area is near the campground and enhances the numerous recreational opportunities provided by the lake, such as boating, skiing, fishing, and swimming. The Corps has done a fine job of making the most of this area, which lies in the center of the Mountain State.

Truth be known, tent campers will like only some of the campground. There are seven loops, and four of them are RV havens. But the first three loops will more than suffice. Pass the check-in station and wind along a road to arrive at Loop A. It has 19 campsites set in a shady hickory-oak forest. It is very hilly, offering vertical relief. The paved pull-ins and tent sites have been leveled, but overall the sites are on the smallish side and a tad close to one another—but they are OK.

Continue just a short distance, passing a fully equipped bathhouse, and come to Loop B. It shares the bathhouse with Loop A. The sites here are much like Loop A, with plenty of shade. Also like Loop A, Loop B has electricity. But the smaller campsites and hilly terrain away from the lake keep out the big rigs.

Beyond this is the Hill Loop. It is situated, as expected, on a hill. It offers a mixture of grass and trees, with some sites more open than others. Most sites have adequate shade. There is no electricity in these eight sites; nor can they be reserved. Nineteen of the 31 sites on Loops A and B can be reserved. Why certain sites were chosen over others to be reserved is a secret known only to the Army Corps of Engineers.

Drive a mile or so farther, top a hill overlooking the pretty lake, and see (ugh!) a sea of RVs down below. There are four camping loops with electricity. They hold a combined 146 big rigs. Stay away from here unless you plan to use the boat ramp, volleyball courts, or horseshoe pit.

Bulltown will fill on most summer weekends, especially holidays. Not surprisingly, Loops A and B are popular because

:: Ratings

BEAUTY: ★ ★ ★ ★
PRIVACY: ★ ★ ★
SPACIOUSNESS: ★ ★ ★
QUIET: ★ ★ ★ ★
SECURITY: ★ ★ ★ ★ ★
CLEANLINESS: ★ ★ ★ ★ ★

:: Key Information

ADDRESS: Bulltown Recreation Area, 2550 S. Main St., Burnsville, WV 26335

OPERATED BY: Army Corps of Engineers

CONTACT: 304-853-2371, **www.lrh .usace.army.mil/missions/recreation /westvirginia/burnsvillelake.aspx;** reservations 877-444-6777, **recreation.gov**

OPEN: Mid-May–Memorial Day

SITES: 8 nonelectric, 196 electric

SITE AMENITIES: Picnic table, fire grate, lantern post

ASSIGNMENT: Reservations accepted but not required

REGISTRATION: At campground

FACILITIES: Hot showers, flush toilets, water spigots, pay phone

PARKING: At campsites only

FEE: $20 per night nonelectric and electric, $26 waterfront electric sites

ELEVATION: 800 feet

RESTRICTIONS:

■ **Pets:** On leash only

■ **Fires:** In fire grates only

■ **Alcohol:** Prohibited

■ **Vehicles:** None

■ **Other:** 14-day stay limit in a 28-day period

they are so shady. You can enjoy a site here nearly any weekday.

While checking in, you notice the Bulltown Historical Area. It is a great tour. There are old structures that represent West Virginia's past. Most were culled from the land that Burnsville Lake now covers. The staff at the interpretive center will show you around, and activities for adults and kids are held here daily. Another part of the historical area is the Battle of Bulltown site. Here, you can see Confederate breastworks and Union fortifications and then learn how and why they fought over the covered bridge spanning the Little Kanawha River. Make the walk around the loop at the Confederate Overlook area.

Also nearby is the Falls Mill Scenic Area. There was once a gristmill at the scenic cascade. It is also a good place to bank-fish if you don't have a boat. Boatless campers can enjoy the nearby swimming beach located on the Little Kanawha arm of the 1,000-acre lake. Boats abound, though, no matter where you are on the water. Many of the arms make for scenic boating, so expect to run into them.

Bikers can enjoy the numerous quiet, paved roads in the large Bulltown area, and hikers can get back to nature on the many trails among the 13,000 land acres. The Whitetail Trail starts near the campground. Get a trail map at the campground check-in station and have a good time.

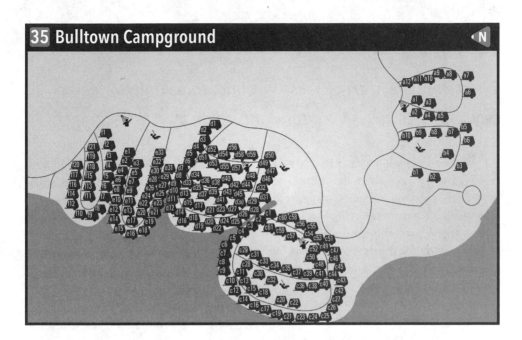

35 Bulltown Campground

:: Getting There

From Exit 67 on I-79 near Flatwoods, head north on US 19 for 11 miles to Millstone Run Road (CR 19/12). Turn left here and drive 1 mile to the left turn into the Bulltown Recreation Area. The campground is dead ahead.

GPS COORDINATES N38° 47.607' W80° 33.623'

Cedar Creek State Park

Located in the heart of West Virginia, this family-oriented, peaceful getaway is used time and again by return campers.

If you are looking for a campground that exudes the peaceful side of life, come here. This state park has a scenic campground tucked away in a mountain valley that allows you to set up your tent and while away the hours, appreciating the fact that you have no agenda. Then you can focus on renewing relationships with your fellow campers, whether they be friends or family. And if the folding chair gets a little old, there are many activities here that reflect West Virginia's commitment to both natural and sporting pursuits.

The campground is situated in the hollow of Big Two Run. Campsites are spread up the creek and allow plenty of privacy and spaciousness. Tent campsites are designated by a T before the campsite number. These sites have no electricity and are sometimes smaller than the others. The area is well groomed. Water spigots are spread throughout the campground. Sycamore, white pine, and crab apple trees provide shade. A mown lawn is the primary understory.

Pass the camp office, located in an authentic log cabin that was moved to the site from Glenville. Campers register here;

:: Ratings

BEAUTY: ★ ★ ★ ★
PRIVACY: ★ ★ ★
SPACIOUSNESS: ★ ★ ★ ★
QUIET: ★ ★ ★ ★
SECURITY: ★ ★ ★ ★ ★
CLEANLINESS: ★ ★ ★ ★ ★

the park staff is available to answer camper questions. Ahead on your left is the group campground, designated by the B campsites, which are used as overflow. The campground generally fills up during the three major holidays and some weekends in summer.

Come to the regular campsites located on both sides of the road, passing the first of three bathhouses. Having three bathhouses in a 65-site campground nearly ensures you will have no wait when cleanup time comes around. There is a small playground here too. The campsites near the first bathhouse have the least shade. Campsite 7 is up a side hollow and is also a trailhead for the Stone Trough Trail.

Cross over Two Run and note some sites on the flat by the creek and other sites on the hill away from the creek. Cross the creek again, and the sites are on the road, left, near the second bathhouse. More dispersed sites continue, with some that are pull-through. The hollow opens up one final time as a side creek comes in from the right. This creates a wide flat where sites at the head of the hollow lie beneath oak and buckeye trees. Here is the third bathhouse. The road turns around. Eleven campsites spoke from the turnaround.

When you decide to get out of your camp chair, you may want to enjoy a cultural pursuit first. On your way to the campground, you undoubtedly noticed the white building on a hill to the left. This is an authentic, one-room schoolhouse that has been restored

:: Key Information

ADDRESS: Cedar Creek State Park, 2947 Cedar Creek Road, Glenville, WV 26351

OPERATED BY: West Virginia State Parks

CONTACT: 304-462-7158, cedarcreeksp.com

OPEN: Early April–mid-October

SITES: 4 nonelectric, 3 electric only, 58 electric and water

SITE AMENITIES: Picnic table, fire grate

ASSIGNMENT: First come, first served, unless reserved

REGISTRATION: By phone or at campground cabin

FACILITIES: Hot showers, flush toilets, phone, laundry

PARKING: At campsites only

FEE: $20 per night nonelectric, $23 water and electric

ELEVATION: 750 feet

RESTRICTIONS:

- **Pets:** On leash only
- **Fires:** In fire grates only
- **Alcohol:** Prohibited
- **Vehicles:** None
- **Other:** 14-day stay limit

and furnished as if the class has gone to lunch on a school day in the 1920s. A park naturalist leads groups through the schoolhouse on Saturdays in the summer.

The swimming pool is a big draw and is open Memorial Day–Labor Day. If you are feeling competitive, try the tennis courts or miniature golf. If you want to fish, there are three ponds covering 10 acres in which you can cast a line. Trout are stocked in spring, and bass, crappie, catfish, and bluegill can be caught year-round. Don't forget the park's namesake, Cedar Creek, where you'll find bass and canoes with anglers fishing for them. The canoes could also be filled with campers enjoying the beauty of the creek when the water is high enough to float a canoe. You must bring your own canoe, but the park rents paddleboats to tool around the fishing ponds.

West Virginia State Parks are known for hiking, and Cedar Creek is no exception. The most popular trails are the Stone Trough and the Park View Trails. The Stone Trough Trail leaves the campground and makes a 2.5-mile loop, which passes a stone watering trough, hand carved from solid rock more than a century ago. The Park View Trail is a challenging 2 miles and passes a rock outcrop, affording views of your natural setting. Add the Cedar Creek Trail to make a loop or if you want to fish from the banks of Cedar Creek. The Two Run Trail follows Two Run up to its source and ties in to the Stone Trough Trail.

The ultimate testimony to a good campground is when campers return year after year. While inquiring about the campground, that was one of the first things park personnel brought up. I knew then that Cedar Creek was a winner.

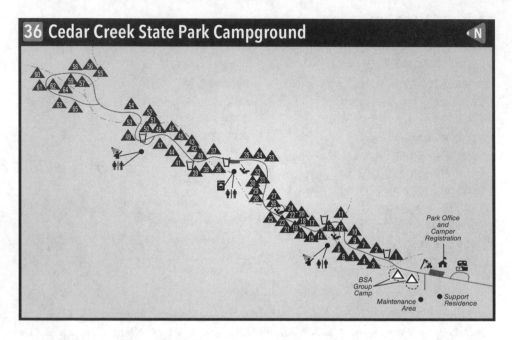

:: Getting There

From Glenville, drive south on US 19 for 4 miles, and turn left on Cedar Creek Road (CR 17). Follow it 4 miles to the state park, which will be on your right.

GPS COORDINATES   N38° 52.486'   W80° 52.494'

37

Coopers Rock State Forest

Camp in the impressive and historic high country near Morgantown, site of West Virginia University.

Coopers Rock is the largest state forest in West Virginia, and it is probably the most studied as well. A good portion of this wooded mountain land is a part of the West Virginia University Research Forest, where students study forestry techniques and their impact on the land and all that grows on it. That is fitting for the flagship state university, which is but a few miles away. While camping here, you can not only check out the natural beauty but also head into Morgantown for a taste of university life, West Virginia style.

Coopers Rock is named for a barrel maker, or cooper, who lived on the mountain in the old days. The rock is an outcropping that overlooks the Cheat River Gorge. This area was once the center of the iron industry in the United States. The Henry Clay Iron Furnace, in the state forest, is a well-preserved example of the iron-making technology of the early 1800s. The timber of the area was used to fire the furnaces. Later, nearly the whole area was logged for wood products. The land has been recovering ever since the state took it over in 1936.

:: Ratings

BEAUTY: ★ ★ ★ ★
PRIVACY: ★ ★ ★
SPACIOUSNESS: ★ ★ ★ ★
QUIET: ★ ★ ★ ★
SECURITY: ★ ★ ★ ★ ★
CLEANLINESS: ★ ★ ★ ★ ★

The 25-site McCollum Campground was added in the 1960s. It is situated on the east side of the main ridge. Even though it is on the side of the ridge, there are many level campsites. The well-wooded camping area with a mostly grassy understory is high quality. You won't find a bad campsite in the entire place.

Begin the teardrop-shaped loop and take the paved high road, passing three campsites; then pass the campground check-in station and the heated bathhouse, which makes showering pleasant on nippy mornings. Then the campground splits into two 11-site loops. The outer loop has more naturally level campsites, which have gravel pull-ins. Evergreens are interspersed throughout the hardwood forest. The campsites face out to the deep woods, where you can see boulders that have tumbled down from the higher ridge.

The campsites on the inner loop have been leveled. The well-shaded sites boast added privacy, due to the site-leveling that's held fast by wooden borders. A couple of pull-through sites will draw RVs. There are good views of the rocky hillside. At a glance, campers will notice that McCollum Campground is well kept and well maintained, even though from late May through August the campground will fill nearly every weekend. Half the sites may be reserved by phone, by mail, or in person from the Friday before Memorial Day through Labor Day. It

:: Key Information

ADDRESS: Coopers Rock State Forest, 61 County Line Drive, Bruceton Mills, WV 26525

OPERATED BY: West Virginia State Parks

CONTACT: 304-594-1561, coopersrockstateforest.com

OPEN: April–October

SITES: 25

SITE AMENITIES: Electricity, picnic table, fire grate, lantern post

ASSIGNMENT: Reservations accepted but not required

REGISTRATION: By phone or at campground check-in station

FACILITIES: Hot showers, flush toilets, water spigots, pay phone

PARKING: At campsites only

FEE: $23 per night

ELEVATION: 2,070 feet

RESTRICTIONS:

■ **Pets:** On leash only

■ **Fires:** In fire grates only

■ **Alcohol:** Prohibited

■ **Vehicles:** None

■ **Other:** 14-day stay limit

will also fill when the West Virginia Mountaineers are playing home football games in the fall.

So what is the draw? Rock climbing is big here. And there are plenty of rock outcroppings, as evidenced by the park's namesake, Coopers Rock, which is easily accessible by a short trail. Other overlooks are at Rock City, whose access trail also starts near Coopers Rock, and Raven Rock, which you can reach by foot from the campground. Another good view can be had from the Sand Springs Fire Tower.

Other trails among the 45 miles of pathways here are over in the University Forest side of the state forest. The Virgin Hemlock Trail passes through a stand of old-growth hemlock trees estimated to be 300 years old.

Get some exercise and a history lesson on the Clay Run Trail. It starts at the campground entrance and goes down 2.5 miles to the historic Henry Clay Iron Furnace. Imagine the bustling scenes here 150 years ago, with the furnace going and men bringing in hand-dug ore, limestone, and hand-cut timber. There were once more than 100 log houses in the vicinity and 200 men employed during the furnace's 12-year run.

There are many other trails. Stop at the Forest Headquarters and get a trail map.

If you want to fish, a 6-acre trout pond is stocked in spring and during October. And if you need a change from the wildlife of the forest, check out the wild life in Morgantown; university towns are always worth a visit, and this one is no exception.

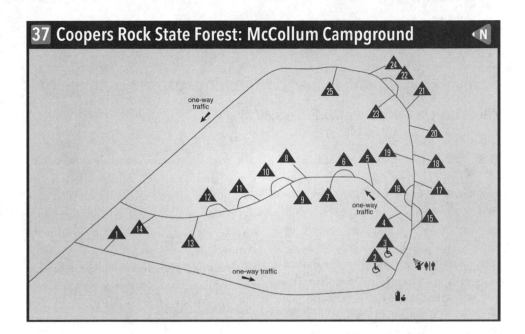

:: Getting There

From Morgantown, take I-68 east to Exit 15, turn right into the state forest, and follow the forest road 1.6 miles to McCollum Campground, which will be on your left.

GPS COORDINATES N39° 38.498' W79° 47.641'

38

Holly River State Park

Many waterfalls and man-made facilities attract campers to the longest campground around.

Webster County is one of the more remote, hilly sections of the state, and that's saying a lot. Holly River State Park is a preserved slice of the county's finest scenery. These hills were carved over time by precipitation. The heavy rainfall in this part of the state results in the dramatic waterfalls for which Holly River State Park is known. Trails lead to the falls and many other natural features of the land.

Beyond the trail system are game courts, a swimming pool, and nature programs. What Holly River should also be known for is having one of the longest campgrounds in the state. More than 80 campsites are stretched alongside Laurel Fork, before the waterway merges with Left Fork Holly River. The long camping area has fair, good, and great campsites. This in one place where you must scout the camping area and pick the campsite that suits you. Warning: There will be some RVs.

Turn into the paved campground road with gravel spur pull-ins. Every campsite has electricity. The first section has campsites that are a little close to the main road. The

oak, hickory, maple, and tulip tree forest has a light understory. Head on down to the next section. Some campsites lie next to a steep hill to your left and are a little less than level. After that, there are many campsites strung right along Laurel Fork. These well-shaded sites have a little rhododendron for added privacy. Continue a good way down the road, where families will be pedaling bikes together, and come to another camping area. Thick hemlock woodland provides year-round shade. The creek is bigger down here, with many campsites along it. Other sites lie across the road, adjacent to the mountainside. In this area, as in other areas of this campground, great campsites sit right alongside the less-than-great ones. The inside of the loop here is less popular.

More camping areas with conveniently placed bathhouses continue. The final camping area has more pines and bigger campsites. In the whole campground, there are only 27 campsites that can be reserved. You should get a reservation before big holidays and on weekends in high summer if you are coming from afar. However, it is also a decent idea to actually pick out your campsite in person if you can, due to the wide variety of desirable and less-than-desirable campsites.

Once here, go waterfall-bagging. There are four major waterfalls at Holly River State Park. You can head to Tecumseh Falls on the Reverie Trail, or Tenskwatawa Falls on a

:: Ratings

BEAUTY: ★ ★ ★
PRIVACY: ★ ★ ★
SPACIOUSNESS: ★ ★ ★
QUIET: ★ ★ ★ ★
SECURITY: ★ ★ ★ ★ ★
CLEANLINESS: ★ ★ ★ ★

:: Key Information

ADDRESS: Holly River State Park, 680 State Park Rd., Hacker Valley, WV 26222

OPERATED BY: West Virginia State Parks

CONTACT: 304-493-6353, hollyriver.com

OPEN: April 15–late November

SITES: 88

SITE AMENITIES: Picnic table, fire grate, electricity

ASSIGNMENT: Reservations accepted but not required

REGISTRATION: By phone or at campground check-in station

FACILITIES: Hot showers, flush toilets, water spigots, coin laundry

PARKING: At campsites only

FEE: $23 per night, 2 primitive sites no charge

ELEVATION: 1,800 feet

RESTRICTIONS:

- **Pets:** On leash only
- **Fires:** In fire grates only
- **Alcohol:** Prohibited
- **Vehicles:** None
- **Other:** 14-day stay limit

spur trail from the Wilderness Trail. Other paths of the 35 miles of trails lead past old homesites and good views. The Potato Knob Trail goes to the Upper Falls and down to the Chute. It also leads up to a large rock outcrop with great views. The Nature Rock Garden Trail is a shorter interpretive trail that has many wildflowers in season. Get a trail map at the park office. Try to see all the falls and climb Potato Knob. It will give you a good idea why all this surrounding vertical ground has so much falling water.

After you are finished with the falls, take a dip in the park pool, which is open Memorial Day–Labor Day. You and your group can also get into a little organized sports competition on the volleyball, basketball, or tennis courts. A park naturalist hosts programs during the summer. Biking the park roads is very popular too.

Sometimes when tent camping, a cookout is a chore. At Holly River you can eat at the park restaurant. This can be handy, as Webster Springs involves a winding drive for its eateries. Full-service stores are located there, should you need to make a supply run. Buckhannon is a good haul to the north. Once at Holly River try to stay put and make the most of your precious tent-camping time.

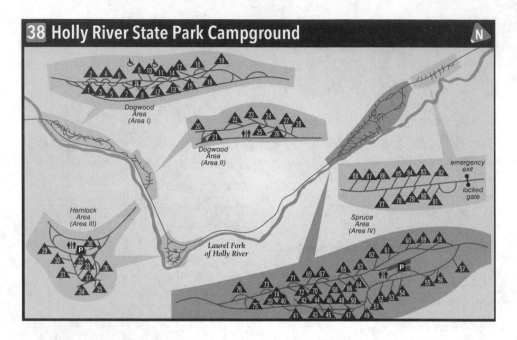

38 Holly River State Park Campground

:: Getting There

From Buckhannon, drive south on WV 20 for 32 miles. Holly River State Park will be on your left.

GPS COORDINATES   N38° 40.019'   W80° 22.110'

39

Pleasant Creek WMA

Pleasant Creek is the campground of choice for tent campers on Tygart Lake. Enjoy Tygart State Park across the water too.

This place should be named Pleasant Campground. Meandering along a ridge, the camping area is laid out with good sites in mind and no worries about cramming too many campers in too little space. Tygart Lake, an Army Corps of Engineers impoundment, is just a half mile away. There is good hiking, fishing, and wildlife-viewing in the Wildlife Management Area. The more developed facilities of Tygart Lake State Park are just a boat ride or short drive away from Pleasant Creek. The campground at Tygart Lake has too many big rigs for me, and the campsites are too hilly. Don't ask me why all the RVs end up there. Plus, Pleasant Creek is a lot cheaper.

Drive down the valley of Pleasant Creek and pass an arm of the lake before entering the campground. Register at the check-in station and pick a campsite. Immediately off to your right is a loop with five spacious sites, a grassy yard with a playground in the center, and a forested perimeter. The first campsite has a covered roof over its picnic table. These campsites aren't overly private but are good for families with kids.

:: Ratings

BEAUTY: ★ ★ ★ ★
PRIVACY: ★ ★ ★ ★
SPACIOUSNESS: ★ ★ ★ ★
QUIET: ★ ★ ★ ★
SECURITY: ★ ★ ★ ★
CLEANLINESS: ★ ★ ★ ★

To your left is a spur road with 13 ultra-spacious campsites. Several sites offer disabled access. The spur road runs along a ridge and is well shaded beneath an oak-hickory forest. The understory consists of smaller trees and brush. Good views of the woods below the ridge add to the campsites here. A pump well and vault toilet are close by. The road ends in a small loop, with a few campsites on the outside of the loop.

The main campground road goes straight ahead from the check-in station and turns right, passing a few secluded sites on the left. More sites overlook a hollow to the right. The road then meanders up a hill, passing another pump well and bathroom area. Campsites are well dispersed and well maintained, and nearly every site lures you to pull your vehicle in. The campground fills on major holiday weekends during the summer. Other than that, campsites should be available.

There are hiking and fishing opportunities here at Pleasant Creek. The Lake Trail leaves the campground from the end of the center spur road and heads down and around the lake. There are many other unnamed trails that thread the area. Get a brochure at the area office. Near the campground is a boat launch. The damlike structure you may see in the water is a waterfowl impoundment. Boaters can angle from the lake for warm-water species. Even if you

:: Key Information

ADDRESS: Pleasant Creek WMA, Route 3, Box 180, Philippi, WV 26416	**REGISTRATION:** Self-registration on-site
OPERATED BY: West Virginia Division of Natural Resources	**FACILITIES:** Pump well, vault toilets
	PARKING: At campsites only
CONTACT: 304-265-1760, **www.wvdnr .gov/hunting/d1wmaareas.shtm#14d1**	**FEE:** $5 per night
	ELEVATION: 1,100 feet
OPEN: Year-round	**RESTRICTIONS:**
SITES: 40	■ **Pets:** On leash only
SITE AMENITIES: Picnic table, fire grate, lantern post	■ **Fires:** In fire grates only
	■ **Alcohol:** Prohibited
ASSIGNMENT: First come, first served; no reservations	■ **Vehicles:** None
	■ **Other:** 14-day stay limit

don't have a boat, you can bank-fish, as I saw many campers do during my visit.

If you want to go to Tygart Lake State Park, head back out to US 119, turn right (north), and drive 6 miles into Grafton. While there, pay a visit to the Grafton National Cemetery, where Civil War veterans are buried. Once at Grafton, follow the signs 3 miles to the state park. You will also pass the visitor center at the Tygart Lake dam, run by the Army Corps of Engineers. Inside are interesting displays about the dam, how it was made, and what it does. The Tygart Dam Trail leaves here and passes by the dam and the park lodge before looping around to intersect the Dogwood Trail and returning to the visitor center. The state park has other trails as well. A park naturalist offers programs during the summer.

A full-scale marina on the lake welcomes boaters and offers boat rentals. Water-skiers, anglers, and even scuba divers will be found on the clear impoundment. There is also a lakeside swimming area with a grassy lawn for sunbathing and game courts. Indulge in these developed facilities, and then return to the rustic and pleasant campground across the lake at Pleasant Creek.

39 Pleasant Creek WMA Campground

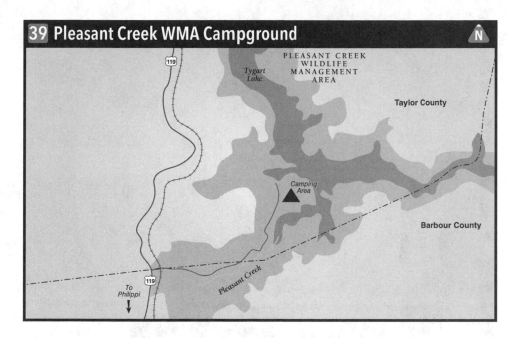

:: Getting There

From Philippi, head north on US 119 for 6 miles and come to Pleasant Creek at the Barbour–Taylor county line. Turn right at the sign for Pleasant Creek, soon pass under a high train trestle, and come to the campground after 3 miles.

GPS COORDINATES   N39° 15.640′   W80° 01.024′

New River Valley

40

Army Camp

The water, land, and history of the New River Gorge await you.

A **name like Army Camp** leads you to believe this location has been camped on for some time. During World War II, the Army Corps of Engineers built bridges over the New River for training. Many of the Corps members were probably here against their will, but you will find no one of that sentiment today. Army Camp is a fine campground run by the National Park Service. It was remodeled and opened for business in the spring of 1999. From here, the trails of Glade Creek, the restored railroad town of Thurmond with its trails, and the water pursuits of the New River are all nearby. Throw in a little auto touring, and you have a great outing in hand.

Army Camp, also known as Camp Prince, is set on a hairpin bend in the New River. First the waterway heads west, then north, and finally back east before resuming its northern course. All around you, the walls of the river gorge rise high overhead. The white noise of McCreery Rapids bubbles in the distance.

The campground is laid out in a loop. The center is mostly clear, as it once was when this locale was farmland. Pass the day-use

area on your right, and immediately come to the bathroom building. The first campsite is on the inside of the loop and is shaded by a lone tree. A river-access trail leads right to the New River. The rest of the riverbank is wooded. The second of five campsites on the inside of the loop comes next.

Pass a second river-access trail on your right, and then come to four nicely wooded campsites on the outside of the loop. These offer views of the gorge yet are well shaded. These sites, like all the others, have excellent tent pads of wood chips. These wood chips allow stakes to be easily driven into them, promote adequate drainage, and make for soft ground and a better night's sleep.

During my stay at Army Camp, a summer storm rolled through. I hurriedly put up my tent as lightning was illuminating the sky in the distance. The tent stakes held fast while the wind whipped and buckets of rain dropped from overhead. I stayed completely dry while thunderclaps echoed through the canyon, creating an impressive yet ominous sound.

Pass two more wooded sites on the outside of the loop. The wooded sites generally are occupied first, though boaters prefer the campsites closest to the water. During the warm months, Army Camp will fill on weekends. Other than that, you should have no trouble getting a campsite, even though they are free.

Around Army Camp you can swim and fish the river. The New is one of the best warm-water fisheries in the state.

:: Ratings

BEAUTY: ★ ★ ★ ★
PRIVACY: ★ ★ ★
SPACIOUSNESS: ★ ★ ★ ★
QUIET: ★ ★ ★ ★
SECURITY: ★ ★ ★ ★
CLEANLINESS: ★ ★ ★ ★

:: Key Information

ADDRESS: Army Camp, P.O. Box 246, Glen Jean, WV 25846

OPERATED BY: National Park Service

CONTACT: 304-465-0508, **nps.gov/neri**

OPEN: Year-round

SITES: 11

SITE AMENITIES: Picnic table, fire grate, lantern post, tent pad

ASSIGNMENT: First come, first served; no reservations

REGISTRATION: Ranger will come by to register you

FACILITIES: Vault toilet; bring water

PARKING: At campsites only

FEE: None

ELEVATION: 1,200 feet

RESTRICTIONS:
- **Pets:** On leash only
- **Fires:** In fire grates only
- **Alcohol:** At campsites only
- **Vehicles:** None
- **Other:** 14-day stay limit in a 28-day period

Smallmouth bass and catfish are angler favorites. A trail leaves the day-use area and follows the river before turning up to McKendree Road. Turn right on the gravel McKendree Road and return to the bridge near Army Camp to make a loop.

McKendree Road is great for auto touring—a high-clearance vehicle makes it a safer ride. From Army Camp it is an approximately 45-minute scenic drive to the old railroad town of Thurmond. A park visitor center occupies the restored train depot. From here, you can tour the old town by foot and learn more about life in the New River Gorge during the early 1900s, when coal fueled explosive growth in West Virginia.

There are several trails in the Thurmond area for hikers and bikers. The Thurmond-Minden Trail follows an old railroad grade along the river, where you cross over five trestles offering great views into the gorge and of Thurmond. The Stone Cliff Trail follows the New River upstream and leads to the Bragg Homestead Site. The Brooklyn–Southside Junction Trail goes through some abandoned mining towns.

And what is a trip to the New River without getting on the river? The section between Hinton and Thurmond is suitable for canoes and kayaks, offering class I–III water. Below Thurmond to the New River Gorge Bridge is big water with class III–V rapids. The rapids are huge here and ideal for rafting. Numerous outfitters operate in the area. Check the park website for a list of licensed outfitters.

After all the fun here, you will find yourself leaving Army Camp against your will.

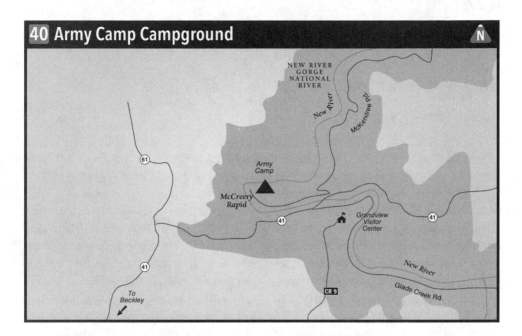

40 Army Camp Campground

NEW RIVER
GORGE
NATIONAL
RIVER

New River

McKendree Rd.

61

Army
Camp

McCreery
Rapid

41

Grandview
Visitor
Center

41

41

New River

Glade Creek Rd.

CR 9

To
Beckley

:: Getting There

From Beckley, take WV 41 north 9 miles toward Prince. Cross the bridge over the
New River, and take your first left. The left turn is just after the bridge crossing.
Follow this road 2 miles and dead-end at Army Camp.

GPS COORDINATES   N37° 51.509′   W81° 05.910′

Babcock State Park

*Stay at Babcock and raft the wild rapids of the
lower New River Gorge.*

Babcock is one of West Virginia's first state parks. It was inaugurated July 1, 1937. The allure of this part of the Appalachian Plateau made it a logical choice. The Civilian Conservation Corps developed the park, and other amenities were added later. The state was right in picking this locale, but little did they know that another primary attraction would develop very nearby. This attraction is the rafting on the lower New River Gorge. Some of the most exciting and certainly most scenic rafting in the country is on the New River. Babcock abuts the New River Gorge National River. Not only can you enjoy the facilities and beauty of Babcock, but you can also hook up with a commercial outfitter from Fayetteville and take on the wild rapids of the New River.

The campground has potential, but I question the location. It is set 2 miles from the main noncamping facilities in the park and is split in two by a road. Granted, the road is little used, but with all the pretty terrain, why put it where it is? Anyway, the site is on a piece of forested plateau land. The main camping area can only be described as an agglomeration of small loops that stay on the most level part of the plateau.

Beyond the check-in station is a white pine, oak, and hickory forest. Pass a few sites under shady hemlocks, and then come to a more open area where oak and hickory dominate overhead. The campsites are normal in size, but privacy is lacking due to the light understory. The second small loop has electric campsites and a bathhouse.

Other sites here are erratically arranged on islands inside gravel roads. The sites are passable, just a little on the open side. Across the road are campsites 41–51. The paved loop is centered in a field with a periphery of woodland. All the sites are on the outside of the loop, allowing shade at some camping spots. Others are wide open. These electric sites are for the big rigs. Stay on the other side of the road.

This campground fills just about every weekend during the summer and is busy all of July. It is also busy during the fall rafting season on the Gauley River, another nearby waterway with very exciting rafting. If you are coming from far away during these periods, reserve a site.

The main draw here is rafting, but the park itself should not be overlooked. There are around 20 miles of hiking and mountain-biking trails. Mountain bikes are available for rent during the summer. The Old Sewell Road leads down to the New River, where you can check out the waters. You can bike a

:: Ratings

BEAUTY: ★ ★ ★
PRIVACY: ★ ★ ★
SPACIOUSNESS: ★ ★ ★ ★
QUIET: ★ ★ ★
SECURITY: ★ ★ ★ ★
CLEANLINESS: ★ ★ ★ ★

:: Key Information

ADDRESS: Babcock State Park, 486 Babcock Road, Clifftop, WV 25831

OPERATED BY: West Virginia State Parks

CONTACT: 304-438-3004, babcocksp.com

OPEN: Mid-April–October

SITES: 24 nonelectric, 28 electric

SITE AMENITIES: Picnic table, fire grate

ASSIGNMENT: First come, first served, unless reserved

REGISTRATION: By phone or at campground registration station

FACILITIES: Hot showers, flush toilets, water spigot, coin laundry

PARKING: At campsites only

FEE: $20 per night nonelectric, $23 electric

ELEVATION: 2,700 feet

RESTRICTIONS:
- **Pets:** On leash only
- **Fires:** In fire rings only
- **Alcohol:** Prohibited
- **Vehicles:** None
- **Other:** 14-day stay limit

12-mile loop by using Old State Road and Old Sewell Road. Hikers can head to scenic overlooks on the Island-in-the-Sky Trail. Manns Creek Gorge Trail also offers views. There is a stable near the campground that has guided horseback rides for adults and pony rides for kids.

You may wish to tour the Old Mill down on Glade Creek. It was reconstructed using pieces of other authentic mills from around the state. Meal is actually ground there today. There are daily tours in the summer and on weekends during the spring and fall.

Boley Lake has 19 acres of fishing. You can also rent paddleboats, rowboats, and canoes. Jump in the swimming pool if you feel like getting wet. There are game courts on-site, and a park naturalist holds programs during the summer.

But most folks come for the rafting. Rapids range up to class V, which means go with a guided outfit for a fun and safe outing. The section of river from Thurmond down to the famous New River Gorge bridge is challenging. From the Sewell area down to the bridge has the most rapids, with names like Millers Folly and Double Z. For a list of licensed outfitters, visit **nps.gov/neri.** I have been down the New during the fall-color season and found it to be one of my favorite outdoor adventures in West Virginia. Your trip will be noteworthy, no matter when you go.

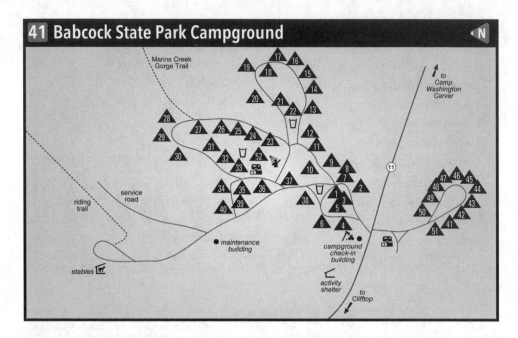

:: Getting There

From Fayetteville, drive north on US 19 to US 60. Head east on US 60 for 10 miles to WV 41 South. Head south on WV 41 for 2 miles and turn right on Clifftop Road. Follow Clifftop Road a short distance to the campground. The registration building will be on your left.

GPS COORDINATES   N38° 00.419′   W80° 56.905′

Bluestone State Park

Bluestone Lake was designed for flood control but is now a recreational haven for water lovers.

The 2,000-acre Bluestone Lake is the focal point of this state park. It is the impoundment of the New and Bluestone Rivers, creating ribbons of water amid steep hollows cut into the land. The free-flowing section of the Bluestone River, above the lake, is a federally designated wild and scenic river. The nearby southern end of the New River Gorge National River offers a couple of good waterfalls for your viewing pleasure. The state park has been developed on the rugged shores of the lake, making for a good place to camp awhile.

Boating and fishing are the top draws, but the hills and hollows make for challenging hiking, with an accent on spring wildflowers and fall colors. A pool, a recreation building with lots of equipment for games, and other man-made amenities keep you busy. So do summer, nature, and park programs.

The campgrounds barely make the grade in comparison to the natural beauty of the area. Meador Campground is more developed and in better shape, but the

development attracts the RV crowd. It does have an eight-site tent area that is OK. Old Mill Campground has potential but could be better developed as a great tent campground. But it is cheap by state park standards.

The Meador Campground is laid out in a rough figure eight along the shore of Bluestone Lake. Much of it is open, but there are decent pockets of white pine, cedar, sycamore, and locust. Drop down on the outer loop and pass along the lake. Six of the campsites are lakeside. Tent campers should be interested in sites 12, 13, and 14. They do not have electricity and are right on the lake. Swing back up the hill and hit the inner loop. The roads are paved, as are the pull-ins. All the well-dispersed campsites here have electricity. The whole setup spells RV.

Nearby is the eight-site tent-camper area, a shady pine grove on a knoll. The slightly sloped sites spoke downhill away from the top of the knoll. There are rock fire rings and picnic tables at the bunched-up campsites. There is a bathroom here, but hot showers are available at Meador Campground.

The Old Mill Campground is set on its own in a flat by the Bluestone River. The campsites are in grassy areas alongside the lake and have just a rock fire ring and a picnic table. The sites near the boat launch are in the open, save for the ring of woodland around the grassy center, where tenters camp. Once you get past campsite 20, the river birch woodland increases and shade

:: Ratings

BEAUTY: ★ ★
PRIVACY: ★ ★
SPACIOUSNESS: ★ ★ ★
QUIET: ★ ★ ★ ★
SECURITY: ★ ★ ★ ★ ★
CLEANLINESS: ★ ★ ★ ★ ★

:: Key Information

ADDRESS: Bluestone State Park, HC 78, Box 3, Hinton, WV 25951

OPERATED BY: West Virginia State Parks

CONTACT: 304-466-2805, **bluestonesp.com**

OPEN: Early May–late October

SITES: 62 nonelectric, 22 electric

SITE AMENITIES: Meador: picnic table, fire grate, lantern post; Old Mill: picnic table, fire ring

ASSIGNMENT: Reservations accepted but not required

REGISTRATION: By phone or at park

FACILITIES: Hot showers, cold showers, flush toilets

PARKING: At campsites only

FEE: Meador: $20 per night nonelectric, $23 electric; Old Mill: $14 electric

ELEVATION: 2,000 feet

RESTRICTIONS:

■ **Pets:** On leash only

■ **Fires:** In fire rings only

■ **Alcohol:** Prohibited

■ **Vehicles:** None

■ **Other:** 14-day stay limit

becomes more abundant. There are 23 riverfront sites.

Make the loop on the gravel road at Old Mill and climb a hill, where the campsites are much more wooded. With a little leveling, these could be great tent sites. Be sure to keep your head on the uphill side of the slope when you try to sleep. The best tent sites are around campsite 37. There is a bathhouse with cold showers for Old Mill campers.

Each of the three camping areas has its pluses and minuses. You will just have to come here and weigh them for yourself. Meador fills on holidays and summer weekends. But you can almost always get a site at Old Mill or the tent area.

By the time you have found a campsite, you will have realized what rugged and beautiful country this is. Most folks enjoy the views from the lake looking up. If you didn't bring your boat, there are boats and canoes for rent at the park marina.

The park pool isn't nearly as big as Bluestone Lake, but it is a good place to cool off.

It is located next to Meador Campground. You can rent croquet or shuffleboard equipment at the recreation building. Look for posted activities led by park personnel. A park naturalist leads programs daily Memorial Day–Labor Day.

The naturalist may coax you onto some park trails. You can trace the former Kanawha Turnpike, a road designated by the old Virginia Assembly in 1838. It was the equivalent of I-77 in those days. This trail lasts a mile and offers lookouts into the mountains. The Overlook Trail also offers vistas. You can take the Big Pine Trail from the Old Mill Campground to connect to these and other pathways.

If you haven't had enough water, drive north on WV 20 to Hinton (where supplies are available) and continue on the west bank of the New River on River Road to check out Brooks Falls and Sandstone Falls. These are major rapids on the New River Gorge National River. It will give you an idea what cut all of these deep hollows around Bluestone.

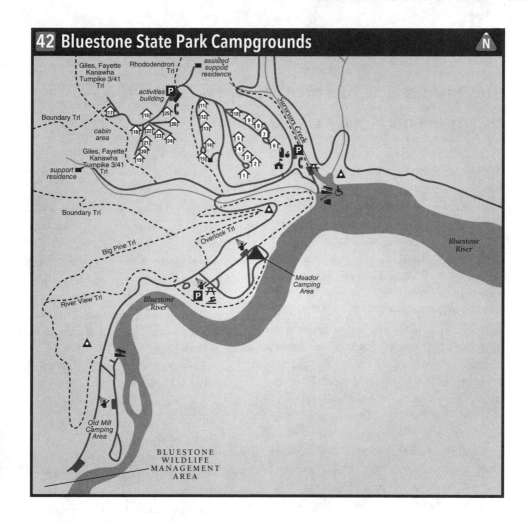

42 Bluestone State Park Campgrounds

:: Getting There

From Hinton, drive south on WV 20 for 5 miles to Bluestone Park Road (CR 20/2). Turn right on Bluestone Park Road and enter the park.

GPS COORDINATES   N37° 36.702′   W80° 56.289′

Brooklyn

This rustic and natural riverside campground is the polar opposite of the Brooklyn in New York.

This campground is located at what was once Brooklyn—a New River mining town, not the Brooklyn of New York. This place is much quieter and more in tune with nature. However, this West Virginia Brooklyn once bustled with miners and their families, who lived and worked in the New River Gorge. Today, you can enjoy a quiet walk-in campground and indulge in the activities abounding nearby. Yet Brooklyn's past remains. Look around for evidence of the coal processing from the Brooklyn Mine hundreds of feet up the gorge wall. There is also loose coal around the parking area.

Here at Brooklyn Campground, you can camp and hike amid history, literally overnighting where a community of miners once dwelled. After driving the final mile on a gravel road, reach the Brooklyn camping area, as well as the trailhead for the Southside Trail. The only drive-up campsite is located just before you turn left to reach the New River. A thick hardwood forest shades this popular campsite. The four walk-in tent sites are stretched out in a row along an old railroad bed about 50 feet above the river. These campsites are level and well shaded.

Each campsite has its own tent area, picnic table, and lantern post. You will notice the stone blocks that were once walls to keep the sloped ground above the campsites in check. I have spent many a night here, and my only complaint is that, unless you are staying at the first walk-in tent site, you have to walk directly beside campsites to reach the farthest ones.

A portable bathroom is located at the walk-in tent parking area. Make sure to bring your own water. Visitors to Brooklyn can use the boat launch to access the New River. I have also used it for swimming and fishing. However, most of the boating action is just downstream at Cunard. This is where commercial outfitters begin exciting trips. The New River is fun for kayakers or rafters, though most novice whitewater aficionados go on rafting trips. Licensed outfitters can be found through the park's website.

Hikers can hit the trail directly from the campground. Take the Southside Trail to the old town of Red Ash. It is a 3.8-mile there-and-back trek. This hike traces the old Chesapeake & Ohio Railroad from the abandoned mining town of Brooklyn along a scenic stretch of the New River to end at another abandoned mining town, Red Ash. View relics of Red Ash, the site of a 1900 mining disaster that killed 46 men. Mother Nature's hand has restored the area to its

:: Ratings

BEAUTY: ★ ★ ★ ★
PRIVACY: ★ ★ ★
SPACIOUSNESS: ★ ★ ★ ★
QUIET: ★ ★ ★ ★
SECURITY: ★ ★ ★
CLEANLINESS: ★ ★ ★

:: Key Information

ADDRESS: Brooklyn Campground, P.O. Box 246, Glen Jean, WV 25846	**FACILITIES:** Vault toilets (bring water)
OPERATED BY: National Park Service	**PARKING:** At campsite and a walk-in parking area
CONTACT: 304-465-0508, **nps.gov/neri**	**FEE:** None
OPEN: Year-round	**ELEVATION:** 1,030 feet
SITES: 4 walk-in tent sites, 1 drive-up tent site	**RESTRICTIONS:**
SITE AMENITIES: Picnic table, fire grate, lantern post	■ **Pets:** On leash only
ASSIGNMENT: First come, first served; no reservations	■ **Fires:** In fire grates only
	■ **Alcohol:** At campsites only
REGISTRATION: Ranger may come by and register you	■ **Vehicles:** None
	■ **Other:** 14-day stay limit in a 28-day period

natural splendor. Revel in the tall trees rising on bluff-pocked hillsides, as well as the roaring rapids of the New River. Or you could visit the Brooklyn Mine located hundreds of feet above. You pass the Brooklyn Mine Trail on the way in. The mostly level walk traverses the upper gorge, where you can soak in occasional views of the wooded canyon stretching to the yon. After a couple of miles, reach the Brooklyn Mine, where you can see the barred-over shaft and mine machinery. After camping, hiking, rafting, fishing, and swimming in the New River, you will be well aware of the differences between West Virginia's Brooklyn and New York's.

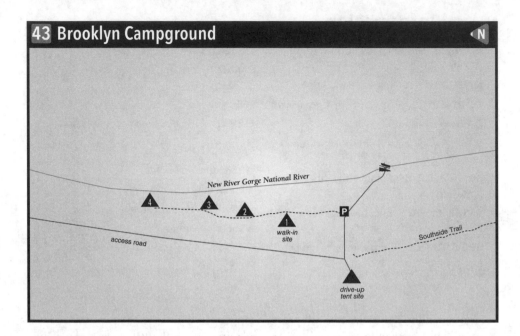

:: Getting There

From US 19 in Oak Hill, take the East Main Street exit. Join WV 16 north and follow it 0.5 mile to Gatewood Road. Turn right on Gatewood Road, WV 14 (look for the national park sign indicating Cunard), and follow it 5.5 miles. Turn right on Cunard Road, CR 9, and follow it 1.7 miles, just past the Cunard Baptist Church; then turn left at the park access road for Cunard. The access road immediately turns left again. Stay with the access road to reach the New River. Once down here, stay right and pass through the commercial boat access area, and then join a gravel road at the far end of the commercial river-access parking. Follow this gravel road 1 mile to dead-end at the trailhead.

GPS COORDINATES   N37° 59.035'   W81° 1.688'

Camp Creek State Park and Forest

If you are traveling down I-77 and need a place to stop, Camp Creek is convenient, but you may find yourself staying a few days and getting off schedule.

Camp Creek State Park and Forest is 5,000 acres of southern West Virginia that are often passed by for other, better-known attractions in the area. Some visitors camp here because it is 2 miles off I-77. There is no doubt that it is a good place to stop on the way to somewhere else, yet it is a worthy destination in its own right. I've spent many a night here. The state park has adequate facilities to keep any tent camper happy. The state forest offers glimpses into a changing landscape that was once farmed but is now scientifically managed for wildlife and timber enhancement. Many old roads, now gated, provide mountain bikers and hikers a chance to enjoy the forest.

There are three campgrounds here: Mash Fork, Blue Jay, and the Double C equestrian campground. The state forest was established in 1953, and the state park was culled from the forest in 1987. After

the park was established, the state saw the need for a more developed, RV-oriented campground, and Mash Fork was born. Tent campers need not bother staying here. Just know that hot showers are available here if you are staying at Blue Jay Campground, which is a mile away, near Campbell Falls. Blue Jay is a shady retreat any tent camper would proudly call home. The equestrian campground is reserved for those with horses.

Drive past the park picnic area and reach Blue Jay, situated beside gurgling Camp Creek. All 13 campsites lie directly along the mountain waterway, beneath a shade-rendering evergreen forest accented with ironwood, also known as American hornbeam or musclewood because the gray bark resembles the sinewy muscles of a human arm or leg. Pioneers, like those who lived in the area before it became a state forest, used this heavy, tough wood for handles, levers, wedges, or land sleds, which were used instead of wagons in irregular, rocky areas where wheels were useless.

Profuse rhododendron provides campsite privacy. The sites are not overly large but are great for those who love being creekside. A couple of water spigots serve the campground; there are two vault toilets up the hill away from Camp Creek. Remember, you

:: Ratings

BEAUTY: ★ ★ ★
PRIVACY: ★ ★ ★
SPACIOUSNESS: ★ ★ ★
QUIET: ★ ★ ★ ★
SECURITY: ★ ★ ★ ★ ★
CLEANLINESS: ★ ★ ★ ★

:: Key Information

ADDRESS: Camp Creek,
2390 Camp Creek Road,
Camp Creek, WV 25820

OPERATED BY: West Virginia State Parks

CONTACT: 304-425-9481,
campcreekstatepark.com

OPEN: Year-round (limited facilities
during cold months)

SITES: 13 nonelectric; 16 electric;
7 water and electric; 3 water, electric,
and sewer; 14 equestrian

SITE AMENITIES: Picnic table, fire grate,
lantern post, wireless Internet at Mash
Fork

ASSIGNMENT: Reservations accepted
but not required

REGISTRATION: By phone, or park
ranger will register you

FACILITIES: Hot showers, flush toilets,
vault toilets, water spigots

PARKING: At campsites only

FEE: $14 nonelectric; $23 electric;
$26 water and electric; $29 water,
electric, and sewer; $21 equestrian

ELEVATION: 2,000 feet

RESTRICTIONS:

■ **Pets:** On leash only

■ **Fires:** In fire grates only

■ **Alcohol:** Prohibited

■ **Vehicles:** 30-foot trailer limit

■ **Other:** 14-day stay limit

must go to Mash Fork Campground to take a shower.

There is no set pattern to when this place fills, other than on summer holidays. Campsite capacity is weather dependent, but you most likely can get a site at Blue Jay during the colder months. I recommend coming here during spring and fall. With little water recreation, it could get uncomfortably hot during the summer.

Just up Camp Creek from the campground is Campbell Falls. The water spills over a series of small ledges and gathers in a large pool. You can enjoy the waterfall after just a brief walk from your campsite. There is another waterfall up Farley Branch, which is a seasonal stream. You can take a foot trail from Blue Jay and walk to these falls, then over toward Mash Fork or down alongside Farley Branch. All these streams can roar at times, and at other times barely trickle or

nearly dry up. But they are usually flowing strongly in springtime, when the creeks get stocked with trout for anglers.

The rest of the trails are in the state forest. These paths follow old mountain roads through the broken woodland. Some of these are old railroad grades from the logging days. The area still has clearings from old farms, as well as clearings designed to enhance wildlife food production.

Use the park map to wind your way around here up creeks and along ridges. Many of the 20 miles of trails are used by mountain bikers. Slower-paced hikers may see wildlife here, most notably beaver, deer, and turkey. Faster-paced hikers may overlook a few things like old farm implements or a grouse. Camp Creek State Park and Forest is often passed by, except by interstate campers. However, other campers, especially mountain bikers, should enjoy this forest too.

44 Camp Creek State Park Campgrounds

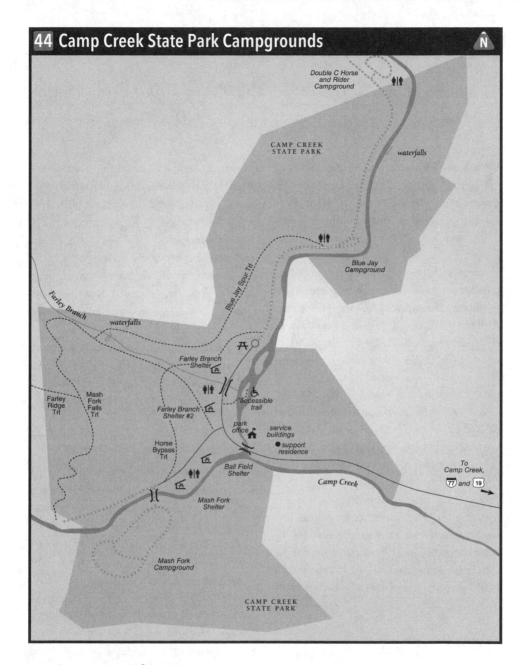

:: Getting There

From Exit 20 on I-77, head south on US 19 a short distance to Camp Creek Road (CR 19/5) and turn right. Follow Camp Creek Road 2 miles to the state park and forest.

GPS COORDINATES   N37° 30.141'   W81° 08.222'

Glade Creek

The campground at Glade Creek is ideally situated for you to enjoy much of the gorgeous scenery at this national river.

The New River Gorge National River is the recreational centerpiece for this part of West Virginia. It is 53 miles of free-flowing water that runs mildly in some places and radically in others, creating paddling opportunities for canoeists, kayakers, and rafters alike. The steep gorge and smaller gorges on side creeks make for natural beauty that can also be enjoyed on foot. And where there is water, there are fish. In the area near the Glade Creek Campground, which is one of the gorge's finer tent campgrounds, fishing is good. And even if you don't catch any, the riverine forest at Glade Creek will raise your spirits. And if that doesn't do it, then remember how much it costs to camp here: nothing.

Drive down to the end of dusty Glade Creek Road and turn into the campground. You are underneath a towering woodland of locust, river birch, buckeye, sycamore, and tulip trees. Other smaller versions of the same trees and more cover the forest floor, creating a dense forest so thick a greenhorn could get turned around inside of 50 yards

:: Ratings

BEAUTY: ★ ★ ★ ★ ★
PRIVACY: ★ ★ ★ ★ ★
SPACIOUSNESS: ★ ★ ★ ★ ★
QUIET: ★ ★ ★ ★
SECURITY: ★ ★ ★
CLEANLINESS: ★ ★ ★ ★

away from his last known spot. Glade Creek tumbles down from the Appalachian Plateau behind you, and the New River rumbles off in the distance.

Take the small road and come to the first place that provides a good sample of the drive-up campsites. It has a pull-through parking area and is culled from the lush growth around it. A picnic table, fire ring, and lantern post adorn the lightly graveled, flat spot. The modern vault toilets are in an elaborate building off to your right. The next campsite has a wooden platform and offers disabled access. The remaining three drive-up sites are much like the first. Any of them would satisfy even the most discriminating tent camper.

The walk-in tent sites are over by the river at the boat launch. Park your car and walk down the sand bar, shaded in river birch and sycamore, and pick one of the six marked campsites. There are great views of the river through the trees. Across the water are the CSX Railroad tracks, which run the length of the entire gorge. You'll find only rock fire rings at the walk-in tent sites because this area occasionally gets flooded by the river and any tables and such would be washed away.

The drawback of this campground is its size. It will fill on nice weekends by Friday night. Come here early Friday if you are a weekend warrior. Luckily, there is a good campground just a few miles away. Just

:: Key Information

ADDRESS: Glade Creek Campground, P.O. Box 246, Glen Jean, WV 25846

OPERATED BY: National Park Service

CONTACT: 304-465-0508, nps.gov/neri

OPEN: Year-round

SITES: 5 drive-up campsites, 6 walk-in tent sites

SITE AMENITIES: Drive-up sites: picnic table, fire ring, lantern post; walk-in sites: fire ring

ASSIGNMENT: First come, first served; no reservations

REGISTRATION: Ranger will come by to register you

FACILITIES: Vault toilets; bring water

PARKING: At campsites or tent-camper parking area

FEE: None

ELEVATION: 1,400 feet

RESTRICTIONS:

■ **Pets:** On leash only

■ **Fires:** In fire rings only

■ **Alcohol:** At campsites only

■ **Vehicles:** None

■ **Other:** 14-day stay limit in a 28-day period

back on Glade Creek Road is the brand-new Grandview Bar Campground. It has 20 drive-up campsites and 15 walk-in tent campsites.

Glade Creek offers good camping, boating, and fishing. A gorgeous set of trails emanate from the campground. A trail leads upriver 0.3 mile to the site of the railroad bridge, whose construction caused the old community of Hamlet to be located here in the first place. The Glade Creek Trail follows an old railroad grade 5 miles through a superscenic mountain vale. There is good trout fishing along this stream. The stocked waterway is catch-and-release for the first 3 miles and catch-and-keep after that. Glade Creek intersects the Kates Falls Trail to view a cascade. The Kates Plateau and Polls Plateau Trails follow old railroad grades. White blazes on trees mark the paths, but be careful, as these trails are hard to follow.

Anglers like to bank-fish or get on the New in johnboats to vie for the numerous smallmouth bass. The swimming is good in

the river, but life jackets are recommended by the park service. There is a solid current.

Another way to get on the New River is by canoe. The section of river from Hinton to Thurmond is class I and II with a few class III rapids. You can and should portage around two rough but pretty spots, Brooks Falls and Sandstone Falls. The 5-mile run from Glade Creek to Grandview Sandbar is a popular and convenient paddle from this campground.

Speaking of Grandview, above you is the Grandview Visitor Center, accessible via Beckley. At Grandview there is a good overlook, interpretive displays, more fun trails, and more park information. Also near here is the Cliffside Amphitheater, featuring dramas such as *The Hatfields and McCoys*, which was played out in real life not too far from here to the southwest. Supplies are available nearby in Beckley. Go ahead and splurge, since the camping at Glade Creek is free.

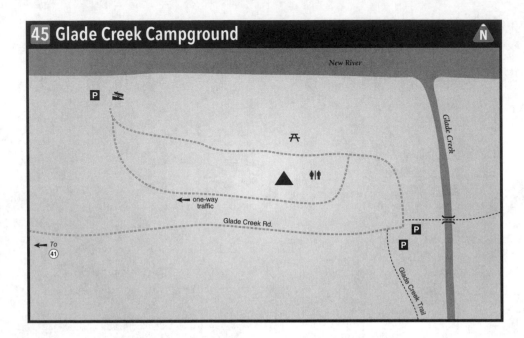

:: Getting There

From Beckley, take WV 41 north 9 miles toward Prince. Turn right on Glade Creek Road just before crossing the bridge over the New River. Follow Glade Creek Road 6 miles to dead-end at Glade Creek Campground.

GPS COORDINATES N37° 49.690′ W81° 00.681′

46

Greenbrier State Forest

The small, attractive campground and slow pace make this a quiet mountain getaway for southeastern West Virginia.

Greenbrier State Forest relies on its natural qualities to attract most visitors. And it should. The campground is nearly ideal in size and setting. The forest itself has activities for the self-motivated outdoors enthusiast, such as hiking and mountain biking, with other outdoor pursuits nearby. There are a few developed facilities, such as a swimming pool. The famed Greenbrier River Trail is just a few miles away, and the Greenbrier River offers canoeing and fishing. West Virginia's most historic cave, Organ Cave, and nearby historic Lewisburg are definitely worth a visit. When you come back from whatever you are doing, the campground will seem like home.

Drive up along Harts Run and come to the campground on your right. Enter an area with five campsites beneath a thick forest of pine, maple, buckeye, oak, and hemlock. The spacious sites have a thick understory for good privacy. A small campground like this one never seems overly busy or crowded, even when it is full.

:: Ratings

BEAUTY: ★ ★ ★ ★
PRIVACY: ★ ★ ★ ★
SPACIOUSNESS: ★ ★ ★ ★
QUIET: ★ ★ ★ ★ ★
SECURITY: ★ ★ ★ ★
CLEANLINESS: ★ ★ ★ ★ ★

Turn right on an upper loop that houses nine campsites. Wooden borders delineate the shady sites. Some are pull-up and others are pull-through. All are desirable, even though those on this upper loop aren't perfectly level. However, tent pads have been installed in bumpier areas.

Leave the upper loop and pass two sites on their own little road. You may have trouble deciding which to choose. The campground fills on Memorial Day weekend and two weekends in August: during the State Fair of West Virginia at Lewisburg and during the Civil War reenactment of the Battle at Dry Creek. Other than that, you should be able to get a campsite anytime, which is surprising, considering the quality and appeal of this campground, plus the few interstate travelers coming off I-64.

Hiking and biking trails at the state forest center around Kates Mountain, which dominates the landscape, and Harts Run, the stream that flows by the campground. The most challenging trek is the Kates Mountain Loop. Head up Rocky Ridge Trail to the top of Kates Mountain. Turn right and then walk along a forest road atop the ridge to drop down to Youngs Nature Trail. Return along Harts Run for an 8-mile circuit. There are overlooks atop Kates Mountain. Other shorter trails exist in the forest, but you may be lured to the Greenbrier River Trail. The southern terminus of this 75-mile rail trail is on the Greenbrier River near Caldwell.

:: Key Information

ADDRESS: Greenbrier State Forest, HC 30, Box 154, Caldwell, WV 24925	**FACILITIES:** Hot showers, flush toilets, water spigots
OPERATED BY: West Virginia State Parks	**PARKING:** At campsites only
CONTACT: 304-536-1944, **greenbriersf.com**	**FEE:** $23
OPEN: April 15–October 31	**ELEVATION:** 2,000 feet
SITES: 16	**RESTRICTIONS:**
SITE AMENITIES: Picnic table, stone fireplace, electricity, wastewater pit	■ **Pets:** On leash only
ASSIGNMENT: Reservations accepted but not required	■ **Fires:** In fireplaces only
	■ **Alcohol:** Prohibited
REGISTRATION: By phone or ranger will come by and register you	■ **Vehicles:** 30-foot trailer limit
	■ **Other:** 14-day stay limit

Mountain bikers love this path, and you may see anglers vying for smallmouth bass.

The Greenbrier is also a good canoe float in season. Contact Outdoor Adventures at (888) 752-9982 or **wvoutdoor adventures.com** for canoe rental and shuttle information.

Lewisburg is a historic destination in its own right. There are many preserved buildings, and the downtown is a federally registered historic district. Lewis Spring, which first brought settlement here, is preserved in a stone springhouse at Andrew Lewis Park. The Old Stone Church, the oldest continuously used church west of the Alleghenies, was built in 1796. The library and a Confederate cemetery are two other interesting sights. Take it all in with a walking tour of downtown.

Another historic walk can be found underground at Organ Cave. Thomas Jefferson visited this cavern, which was used extensively by the Confederates for saltpeter (used in making gunpowder). Take the regular tour, or bring your old clothes for a lesser traveled, down-and-dirty wild cave tour. There are brochures for Organ Cave at the state forest office. After this little adventure, you will certainly appreciate the showers back at Greenbrier State Forest.

46 Greenbrier State Forest Campground

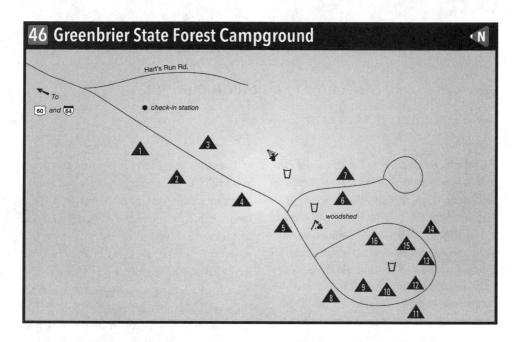

:: Getting There

From Lewisburg, drive east on I-64 for 6 miles to Exit 175. Turn right onto CR 60/14 and drive south 2 miles to Greenbrier State Forest.

GPS COORDINATES N37° 44.575' W80° 21.476'

47

Moncove Lake State Park

Moncove Lake is situated in a quiet mountain valley off the beaten path.

Moncove Lake lies at the southeasternmost edge of West Virginia's ridge and valley country, in the Sweet Springs Valley. In 1959, Devils Creek was dammed to make this mountain impoundment, which provides 144 acres of clear water ready for anglers and small boaters. Middle Mountain and Cove Mountain form scenic bastions overlooking Moncove Lake. Add a little development and a campground with one loop especially suited to tent camping and you have a true recreation destination.

Things don't get hopping at Moncove Lake until Memorial Day, when the campers really roll in, to enjoy not only the lake but also the swimming pool. The pool is set on the shores of Moncove Lake, offering a great view with all the conveniences of swimming in a man-made environment.

The campground has two loops. The right loop, built on a partially forested slight slope, is bordered by two seasonal streams. This loop runs away from the lake, with the upper part shaded by pine trees. Its best attribute is a lake view from some of the campsites. That is because this loop is awfully open, though occasional maple trees dot the lower part. It also has electricity, which attracts the RVs that make it to Moncove. If you have any questions, the park office is oddly located in this loop. This may be the only park office I have seen in the middle of a campground loop. You will find the park staff very relaxed.

The left loop is much better suited to tent camping. Pass from the open area into a hickory/oak forest that's thickly canopied overhead and perched on a hilly area. The hills are not a detriment because the campsites have been leveled, and the leveling adds to the scenery. White pine is more prevalent farther along the loop. The sites are average size and spread well apart. The loop drops down along Devils Creek, the outflow of Moncove Lake. The five campsites strung out along Devils Creek are among the finest in the park. A water spigot and bathhouse are at the end of the loop.

Water recreation is the name of the game here. Moncove Lake holds trout, bass, bluegill, and catfish. People bank-fish from the dam and at designated lake access areas. Others picnic along the lake. You'll find johnboats and paddleboats for rent, and if you bring your own boat, remember that no motors over 5 horsepower are allowed.

Younger kids will enjoy the new pool built on the shores of Moncove Lake. Adults may want to take a dip after a hike on one

:: Ratings

BEAUTY: ★ ★ ★ ★
PRIVACY: ★ ★ ★
SPACIOUSNESS: ★ ★ ★
QUIET: ★ ★ ★
SECURITY: ★ ★ ★ ★ ★
CLEANLINESS: ★ ★ ★ ★ ★

:: Key Information

ADDRESS: Moncove Lake State Park, Route 4, Box 73-A, Gap Mills, WV 24941

OPERATED BY: West Virginia State Parks

CONTACT: 304-772-3450, **moncovelakestatepark.com**

OPEN: April–November

SITES: 23 nonelectric, 25 electric

SITE AMENITIES: Picnic table, fire grate

ASSIGNMENT: First come, first served; no reservations

REGISTRATION: At campground check-in station

FACILITIES: Hot showers, flush toilets, water spigots

PARKING: At campsites only

FEE: $20 per night nonelectric, $23 electric

ELEVATION: 2,500 feet

RESTRICTIONS:

■ **Pets:** On leash only

■ **Fires:** In fire grates only

■ **Alcohol:** Prohibited

■ **Vehicles:** None

■ **Boats:** Motors 5 horsepower and under

■ **Other:** 14-day stay limit

of the park's many trails. The Devils Creek Trail leaves the left loop and parallels Devils Creek. From here, you can turn right and make a loop with Diamond Hollow Trail, or loop around on the Roxalia Springs Trail. Organized sports are played on the park's ball field.

This is an easygoing park where relaxing, maybe watching a bobber at the end of your fishing line, is the most popular pastime. However, there are other attractions, such as the Greenbrier River and the Greenbrier River Rail Trail, to lure hikers, mountain bikers, and paddlers. You can fish the Greenbrier River for bass or take a relaxed float in a canoe. Organ Cave and Lost World Caverns offer underground tours, with a surprising amount of human history thrown in. When you come here, just make sure you camp in the good loop.

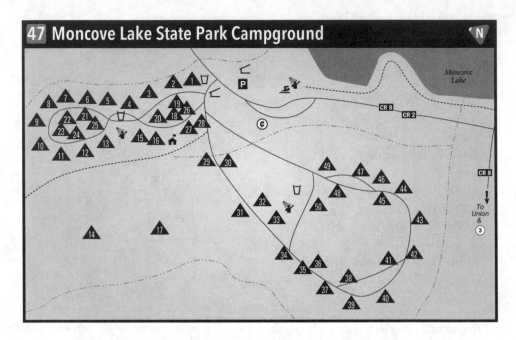

47 Moncove Lake State Park Campground

:: Getting There

From Union, drive east on WV 3 for 9 miles to CR 8. Turn left on CR 8 and follow it 6 miles to the state park, which will be on your left.

GPS COORDINATES   N37° 37.063′   W80° 21.306′

Ohio River Valley

48

Lewis Wetzel WMA

The trail-laced terrain here is as rugged as the legendary
West Virginia pioneer for whom it was named.

Lewis Wetzel worked his way west through old Virginia in the late 1700s. It was a rough place—American Indians still freely roamed the land that later became West Virginia. Day-to-day living was dangerous. But this pioneer exemplified the courage and fortitude to survive in the wilderness he later made home. Wetzel County is home to this 12,000-acre wildlife management area, named in the pioneer's honor. You will find this place no longer as wild as Wetzel did, but it is a good place to camp, fish, and hike.

The campground is in a scenic setting and boasts more than 27 miles of trails, in addition to numerous jeep roads. The area, with elevations ranging from 700 to 1,500 feet, is managed for wildlife; you may see a critter or two. Be apprised this is a hunting zone. Call ahead to check dates so you can safely roam this pretty and rugged slice of northwest West Virginia.

After you drive up Buffalo Run, a side road splits off to the left. Putter through the woods, cross a bridge over a stream, and then come to a clearing surrounded by steep ridges on both sides. This is the confluence of Buffalo Run and Horse Run. The clearing is thick with green grass. Buffalo Run flows on your right. The campground begins. Pass the vault toilets and you'll find a string of campsites backed against the wooded creek. The campsites themselves are in the open, for the most part. This could create a shade problem, but it does open up the view.

Wooden posts delineate the campsites. The sites are far apart, but the openness of the campground cuts down on camper privacy. Bring the big tent—spaciousness is no problem. Head on up to the top of the road; a turnaround houses some really large sites.

Campsites are available any time of the year, except maybe the opening day of deer season. This may be a good place to come in winter to practice your cold-weather camping skills. Late spring could be good too. High summer may be hot. Just call ahead to check for hunting dates.

Lewis Wetzel has some of the best hiking in this part of the state. The fishing isn't bad either. Trout are stocked in spring along the South Fork and North Fork Fishing Creek. South Fork Fishing Creek is known for its smallmouth bass. Good angling gave Fishing Creek its name. Anywhere along the road near Jacksonburg has good small-mouth populations.

The trails are what will keep you coming back. They run up the hollows and along the ridges. I suggest hiking early or late to

:: Ratings

BEAUTY: ★ ★ ★ ★
PRIVACY: ★ ★
SPACIOUSNESS: ★ ★ ★ ★ ★
QUIET: ★ ★ ★ ★
SECURITY: ★ ★ ★ ★
CLEANLINESS: ★ ★ ★ ★

:: Key Information

ADDRESS: Lewis Wetzel WMA, HC 62, Box 8, Jacksonburg, WV 26377

OPERATED BY: West Virginia Division of Natural Resources

CONTACT: 304-889-3497, **www.wvdnr .gov/hunting/d1wmaareas.shtm**

OPEN: Year-round

SITES: 20

SITE AMENITIES: Picnic table, fire grate

ASSIGNMENT: First come, first served; no reservations

REGISTRATION: Self-registration on-site

FACILITIES: Vault toilets; bring water

PARKING: At campsites only

FEE: $5 per night

ELEVATION: 1,150 feet

RESTRICTIONS:

- **Pets:** On leash only
- **Fires:** In fire grates only
- **Alcohol:** At campsites only
- **Vehicles:** None
- **Other:** 14-day stay limit

maximize your chances of wildlife viewing. The Horse Run Trail leaves from just below the campground and runs a mile to the High Knob Trail. You can turn left here and follow the Hart Trail to the Lesin Run Trail and down to Buffalo Run for a 3-mile loop.

For a longer loop, keep going on the High Knob Trail all the way to the Hiles Run Trail. Then drop down to Buffalo Run Road and return to the campground for a 7-mile circuit. Many other trails spur off the High Knob Trail for other loops. Get a trail map

from the manager's office, which is conveniently located just down the road from the campground. This is also where the Locust Trail starts and makes a 2.5-mile loop into the ridges. You will notice there are numerous closed jeep roads on the west side of the area that are ripe for walking or biking.

Yet another trail leaves the campground and heads straight up Buffalo Run, with a side trail going up Meathouse Branch. I wonder what's up there? I guess I'll have to come back and find out.

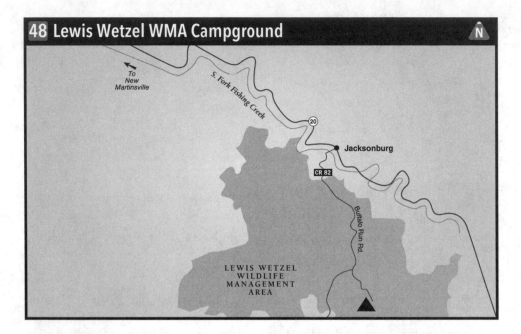

48 Lewis Wetzel WMA Campground

:: Getting There

From New Martinsville, drive 23 miles east on WV 20 to the town of Jacksonburg. Turn right on Buffalo Run Road (CR 82) and cross South Fork Fishing Creek. Lewis Wetzel Wildlife Management Area is dead ahead.

GPS COORDINATES   N39° 28.482′   W80° 37.531′

49

North Bend State Park

The nationally acclaimed North Bend Rail Trail is the centerpiece of this park.

North Bend State Park was here before the North Bend Rail Trail, but now the North Bend Rail Trail gets all the notoriety. This is one of the nation's most scenic and successful rail-to-trail conversions. The north bend referred to is a significant turn in the North Fork of Hughes River, which the trail follows and the park abuts. The rail-to-trail conversion began in 1989 and currently covers more than 70 miles, running from near Parkersburg 27 miles to North Bend State Park and then east another 43 miles to Wolf Summit. North Bend is an excellent place not only to enjoy this nationally acclaimed trail but also for a little tent camping and more.

But just as the old Baltimore and Ohio Railroad is being changed from rail to trail, so is North Bend State Park changing. Acquired land and park expansion have led to an additional campground, a lake with a beach, a new swimming pool, and equestrian trails, making North Bend even better.

The 49-site River Run Campground was the original. Wind your way through the park and end up at River Run, on the banks of the North Fork of Hughes River. The first set of sites between the river and a fishing pond are shaded by sycamores and other creek-loving trees. You have your choice of camping along still or moving water. The understory is mowed grass.

Pass by the pond and come to the campground check-in station/store. Fishing equipment and a few supplies are here. A spur road near the check-in station has more tent campsites. The six pondside sites are great but are a little in the open. However, you can throw in a fishing line right from your tent. The sites away from the pond are on a slope and should be avoided.

Around the corner behind a hill are the electric sites. The loop follows a bend in the North Fork of Hughes River. Twelve of the campsites are riverside. Some of the sites in the center of the loop are too open. Pass the bathhouse, and there are more sites with adequate shade. This area is currently the domain of RVs because of the electricity. Some of these sites can be reserved. Overall, River Run campground is appealing.

Cokeley Campground is situated on a bend in the park lake, completely separated from River Run Campground. Laid out in a classic loop, the electrified campground attracts bigger rigs. Half of the 28 sites front the lake. A bathhouse and play area center the loop. These newer sites will get snapped up, but nonelectric sites are generally available, save for summer holiday weekends.

:: Ratings

BEAUTY: ★ ★ ★
PRIVACY: ★ ★ ★
SPACIOUSNESS: ★ ★ ★ ★
QUIET: ★ ★ ★ ★
SECURITY: ★ ★ ★ ★
CLEANLINESS: ★ ★ ★ ★

:: Key Information

ADDRESS: North Bend State Park, 202 North Bend Park Road, Cairo, WV 26337

OPERATED BY: West Virginia State Parks

CONTACT: 304-643-2931, northbendsp.com

OPEN: Mid-April–November

SITES: 23 nonelectric, 54 electric

SITE AMENITIES: Picnic table, fire grate, stand-up grill, some lantern posts

ASSIGNMENT: Reservations accepted but not required

REGISTRATION: By phone or at campground check-in station

FACILITIES: Hot showers, flush toilets, pay phone, laundry

PARKING: At campsites only

FEE: $15 per night nonelectric, $19 electric

ELEVATION: 850 feet

RESTRICTIONS:

■ **Pets:** On leash only

■ **Fires:** In fire grates only

■ **Alcohol:** Prohibited

■ **Vehicles:** None

■ **Other:** 14-day stay limit

The park trailhead for the North Bend Rail Trail is located near River Run Campground. Bikers enjoy the varied scenery on this path, from valleys to rural communities. Head east on the trail to traverse one of the 12 tunnels and 32 bridges that were once part of the B & O Railroad, constructed from 1853 to 1857. The rail bed has been made more user-friendly. There are three tunnels in the park vicinity. Bring your bike, or rent one at the campground check-in station. Hikers and horseback riders are welcome too.

The park has other standard trails as well. Check out the large rock formation on the Castle Rock Trail. The Giant Pine Trail heads through a grove of white pines. The Hibbs Cemetery Trail leaves the campground and climbs steeply to the Hibbs Family Cemetery. The Nature Trail is the

park's most challenging. It forms a 4.5-mile loop and traverses the varied terrain of the park, including that along the Hughes River and up on rock outcrops of the high ridges. Don't be surprised if you see a deer. North Bend State Park is known for an abundance of does and bucks. Tired of walking? Fish in the pond, lake, or river. Canoeing the North Fork Hughes River is popular too.

The developed areas include tennis, volleyball, and miniature golf, all located near the North Bend Lodge, where you can get a good meal if you tire of roasting hot dogs over the fire. Cool off in the park swimming pool.

The North Bend Rail Trail will probably always overshadow North Bend State Park, but the park does provide a good base camp to enjoy the rail trail and other sights of the park and beyond.

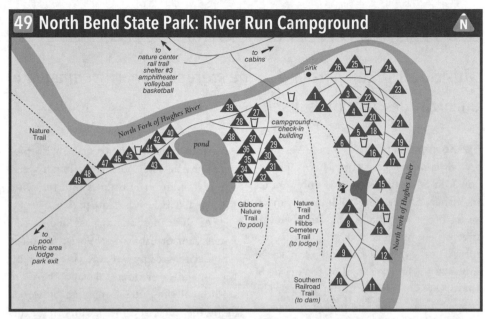

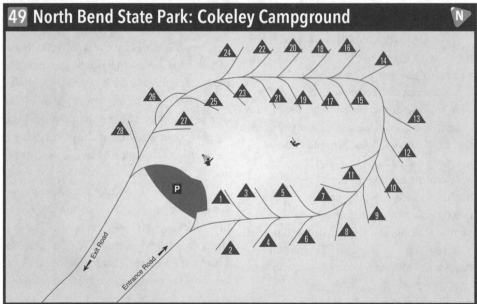

:: Getting There

From downtown Harrisville, drive west on Main Street (CR 5) 4 miles and you will drive straight into the state park. The turn into the park and the campground will be on your right.

GPS COORDINATES   N39° 13.512′   W81° 06.280′

50

Tomlinson Run State Park

This ridgetop campground in the state's northern peninsula is a worthy destination in itself.

The northern peninsula of West Virginia is unique. And where Tomlinson Run State Park lies, it is only 5 miles in either direction to Ohio or Pennsylvania. West Virginia is lucky to have this pretty piece of our country. Tomlinson Run forms a valley where steep ridges make for mountainous terrain. And on top of one of these ridges is the park's campground. The heavily forested high ground gives a sense of being on top of the world, though the elevation is only 1,200 feet.

Actually, all around you is a fine state park, with some development tastefully added to the natural beauty of the area. Trails, a lake, fishing ponds, and a wilderness area are mixed with a huge pool, game courts, and picnic areas. So pack your tent and head on up to West Virginia's northernmost campground.

Wind your way up the ridge and come to the wooded camping area that splits in two directions along the ridge and is divided by the campground check-in station. To your left, south, is the Chief Big Foot Camping Area. This area is named after a 7-foot

American Indian who struggled with pioneers in the late 1700s, meeting his end where Tomlinson Run flows into the Ohio River, a mile below the state park.

At the campground, pass one of this park's camper cabins and yurts, for those who desire to camp but still can't part with the amenities of home. Beyond these are traditional campsites, separated by woods along the ridge, and the bathhouse for this area. A campground host is stationed near here for safety and assistance.

Veer right around the small loop. Some of the sites are pull-through. Just past the loop is a spur road with the most secluded sites. These are among the 10 campsites that can be reserved. The red maple– and sugar maple–dominated forest drops off sharply below the campground, leaving a lot of sky above.

The Chief Logan Camping Area swings around the opposite side of the ridge. The first four campsites are nonelectric. The spacious sites are even more dispersed than the Chief Big Foot Area. Past the bathhouse, the gently rolling ridge dips down but soon levels again. A couple of sites are pull-through. A small turnaround area features five nonelectric sites that are the park's best. The ridge drops off sharply here too.

Tomlinson Run can be busy. It fills nearly every weekend during high summer. Make reservations if you are coming from a long distance. It is sure to fill on big summer

:: Ratings

BEAUTY: ★ ★ ★ ★
PRIVACY: ★ ★ ★ ★
SPACIOUSNESS: ★ ★ ★
QUIET: ★ ★ ★ ★ ★
SECURITY: ★ ★ ★ ★
CLEANLINESS: ★ ★ ★ ★ ★

:: Key Information

ADDRESS: Tomlinson Run State Park, 84 Osage Road, New Manchester, WV 26056

OPERATED BY: West Virginia State Parks

CONTACT: 304-564-3651, tomlinsonrunsp.com

OPEN: April 1–October 31

SITES: 15 nonelectric, 39 electric

SITE AMENITIES: Picnic table, fire grate, lantern post

ASSIGNMENT: Reservations accepted but not required

REGISTRATION: By phone or at campground check-in station

FACILITIES: Hot showers, flush toilets, water spigot, pay phone, coin laundry

PARKING: At campsites only

FEE: $20 per night nonelectric, $24 electric, $30 Rent-a-Camp

ELEVATION: 1,200 feet

RESTRICTIONS:

■ **Pets:** On leash only

■ **Fires:** In fire grates only

■ **Alcohol:** Prohibited

■ **Vehicles:** None

■ **Other:** 14-day stay limit

holidays. Once here, be sure to store your food. The raccoons are stealthy and persistent, and they will eat your food, unless it is properly put away.

Tomlinson Run is known for its swimming pool, which can accommodate 1,600 people. It also has a 182-foot figure-eight waterslide. Kids, have fun. Tennis courts and horseshoe pits are nearby. The park also went big when building its miniature-golf course.

There is other water besides the big pool. Four ponds are stocked with bass and bluegill. The North Fork and South Fork of Tomlinson Run have been dammed to form Tomlinson Run Lake. This impoundment also features fishing for bass, bluegill, channel catfish, and trout during the spring months. Rowboats and paddleboats are available for rent.

The valleys and ridges are striking, as Tomlinson Run drops more than 100 feet per mile en route to the Ohio River. Campers can enjoy many of the trails here by mountain bike or foot. The Poe Trail leaves the campground and heads to the fishing ponds or down to the South Fork to intersect the Big Foot Trail. Follow the Big Foot Trail along the lake to the new Half King Trail, and return to the campground.

The prettiest location may be the park wilderness area. Follow the Laurel Trail down to the White Oak Trail and see the spring wildflowers, deep woods, and overhanging cliffs. Fall is especially colorful. It was just below this area that the settlers tracked Chief Big Foot by his namesake footprints, which led to the encounter on the banks of the Ohio between Andrew Poe and Chief Big Foot. Now the times have changed, and the story is a West Virginia legend. Make some memories of your own up here in the northern panhandle.

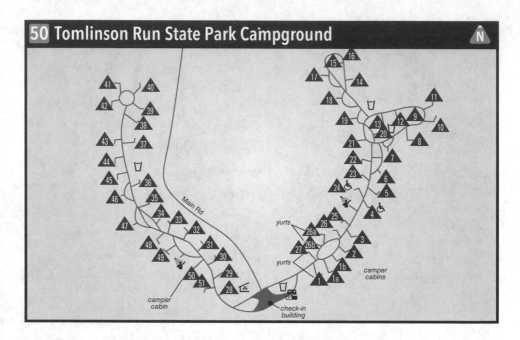

:: Getting There

From New Cumberland, take WV 2 north to WV 8. Drive east on WV 8 north 3 miles to the state park entrance, which will be on your left.

GPS COORDINATES   N40° 32.878'   W80° 34.768'

APPENDIX A

● ● ● ● ● ● ● ● ● ● ● ● ● ● ● ● ● ● ● ●

Camping Equipment Checklist

Except for the large and bulky items on this list, I keep a plastic storage container full of the essentials for car camping so they're ready to go when I am. I make a last-minute check of the inventory, resupply anything that's low or missing, and away I go.

COOKING UTENSILS

Bottle opener

Bottles of salt, pepper, spices, sugar, cooking oil, and maple syrup in water-proof, spillproof containers

Can opener

Corkscrew

Cups (plastic or tin)

Dish soap (biodegradable), sponge, and towel

Flatware

Food of your choice

Frying pan, spatula

Fuel for stove

Lighter, matches in water-proof container

Plates

Pocketknife

Fire starter

Pot with lid

Stove

Aluminum foil

Wooden spoon

FIRST AID KIT

Band-Aids

First-aid cream

Gauze pads

Aspirin

Insect repellent

Moleskin

Sunscreen/lip balm

Tape (waterproof adhesive)

Diphenhydramine (Benadryl)

SLEEPING GEAR

Pillow

Sleeping bag

Sleeping pad (inflatable or insulated)

Tent with ground tarp and rainfly

MISCELLANEOUS

Bath soap (biodegradable), washcloth, and towel

Camp chair

Candles

Cooler

Deck of cards

Flashlight/headlamp

Paper towels

Plastic zip-top bags

Sunglasses

Toilet paper

Water bottle

Wool blanket

OPTIONAL

Barbecue grill

Binoculars

Field guides on bird, plant, and wildlife identification

Fishing rod and tackle

GPS

Lantern

Maps (road, trail, topographic; paper or downloaded)

APPENDIX B

● ●

Sources of Information

MONONGAHELA NATIONAL FOREST
200 Sycamore St.
Elkins, WV 26241
304-636-1800; **www.fs.usda.gov/mnf**

WEST VIRGINIA DEPARTMENT OF TOURISM
Capitol Complex, Bldg. 6, Room 525
Charleston, WV 25305-0311
800-225-5982; **wvtourism.com**

WEST VIRGINIA STATE PARKS
324 Fourth Ave.
South Charleston, WV 25303
304-558-2764

WEST VIRGINIA DIVISION OF NATURAL RESOURCES
324 Fourth Ave., Bldg. 74
South Charleston, WV 25303
304-558-2754; **wvdnr.gov**

NEW RIVER GORGE NATIONAL RIVER
P.O. Box 246
Glen Jean, WV 25846
304-465-0508; **nps.gov/neri**

U.S. ARMY CORPS OF ENGINEERS
Recreation Resources Branch
502 Eighth St.
Huntington, WV 25701
304-399-5211; **www.lrh.usace.army.mil**

GEORGE WASHINGTON NATIONAL FOREST
109 Molineau Road
Edinburgh, VA 22834
540-984-4101; **www.fs.usda.gov/mnf**

INDEX

● ●

ABOUT THE AUTHOR

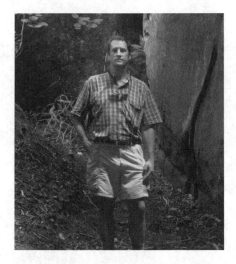

Johnny Molloy is an outdoors writer based in Johnson City, Tennessee. His outdoor life began on a backpacking trip into the Great Smoky Mountains National Park. That first trip, though a disaster, unleashed an innate love of the outdoors that has led to his spending more than 150 nights per year in the wild over the past 25 years, tent camping, backpacking, and canoe camping throughout the country.

After graduating from the University of Tennessee with a degree in economics, he continued to spend an ever-increasing amount of time in natural places, becoming more skilled in the outdoor realm. Friends enjoyed his adventure stories, and one even suggested he write a book. Soon he was parlaying his love of the outdoors into an occupation.

The results of his efforts are more than 55 books and guides, including hiking guides to West Virginia's Monongahela National Forest and the New River Gorge.

Molloy continues to write and travel extensively to all four corners of the United States, participating in a variety of outdoor pursuits. For his latest updates, check out his website at **johnnymolloy.com.**

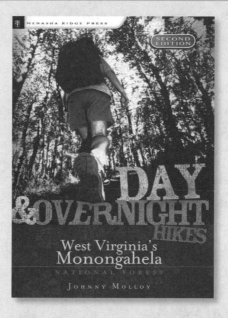

DEAR CUSTOMERS AND FRIENDS,

SUPPORTING YOUR INTEREST IN OUTDOOR ADVENTURE, travel, and an active lifestyle is central to our operations, from the authors we choose to the locations we detail to the way we design our books. Menasha Ridge Press was incorporated in 1982 by a group of veteran outdoorsmen and professional outfitters. For many years now, we've specialized in creating books that benefit the outdoors enthusiast.

Almost immediately, Menasha Ridge Press earned a reputation for revolutionizing outdoors- and travel-guidebook publishing. For such activities as canoeing, kayaking, hiking, backpacking, and mountain biking, we established new standards of quality that transformed the whole genre, resulting in outdoor-recreation guides of great sophistication and solid content. Menasha Ridge continues to be outdoor publishing's greatest innovator.

The folks at Menasha Ridge Press are as at home on a white-water river or mountain trail as they are editing a manuscript. The books we build for you are the best they can be, because we're responding to your needs. Plus, we use and depend on them ourselves.

We look forward to seeing you on the river or the trail. If you'd like to contact us directly, join in at www.trekalong.com or visit us at www.menasharidge.com. We thank you for your interest in our books and the natural world around us all.

SAFE TRAVELS,

Bob Sehlinger

BOB SEHLINGER
PUBLISHER